Ethical issues in palliative care
reflections and considerations

Edited by Patricia Webb

HOCHLAND & HOCHLAND LTD

Published by Hochland & Hochland Ltd,
The University Precinct, Oxford Road, Manchester M13 9QA.

ISBN 1 898507 27 9

A catalogue record for this book is available from the British Library.

Printed in Scotland by Bell & Bain Ltd.

Contents

Foreword

This book is not meant to be a definitive text about ethics in palliative care. It is intentionally a collection of reflections and ideas from a variety of people who either work in palliative care, teach aspects of it, are researching aspects of it, come into regular contact with patients and families who have a progressive, life-limiting illness or all of the above. All of us who have contributed to this book acknowledge the difficulties in making ethical decisions in the everyday practice of palliative care. Over the years we have tried to help each other in a variety of ways, not least by discussing some of the thorny issues for clinicians and the patients they work with. We have included brief information about the experience and specialties of each author at the beginning of each chapter.

As the specialty of palliative care becomes more sophisticated and the illness trajectories of patients become longer, the ethical issues change. They also change because society changes all the time in its views, beliefs and degree of involvement in decisions related to health and ill-health.

It is frequently claimed that there are no finite or absolute answers to ethical dilemmas. The contributors to this book have therefore raised questions, debated them, on some occasions partly given their own opinion but, more helpfully, they have left the reader with the tools to think in a more structured and rational way about the problems.

Many of the issues covered in this book are raised regularly by the health professionals of tomorrow – the undergraduates planning to work in healthcare. Others have been hotly debated by current practitioners working each day in a specialist palliative care setting or those who work with palliative care patients in the generalist settings where the majority are housed.

All of the contributors to this book are well used to teaching health professionals, or students of those professional disciplines in mixed groups. In our collective experience this is by far the most useful way of teasing out some of these ethical dilemmas. They of course do so from their own professional stance but with the recognition that theirs is not the only contribution. To say that we all need all of the help that we can muster would not be exaggerating the point. If patients and families are to be helped to understand what is happening to them and to be given a balanced view of some of the difficult decisions that they will have to make in their contract or alliance with those caring for them, they at least need to know that these ethical issues are taught, thought about and considered by all those with some expertise. This may be the moral philosopher, the doctor, the nurse, the physiotherapist or whoever. Combining the expertise has in our view been helpful.

We very much hope that you will be challenged, helped, or even outraged – if it enables us all to give a greater service to the patients with whom we have contact or those who work with them.

Patricia Webb

CHAPTER ONE

Why is the study of ethics important?

Patricia Webb

Patricia Webb is a Principal Lecturer in Palliative Care at St George's Hospital Medical School and Trinity Hospice, London. Having initially trained as a nurse and become fascinated with cancer, she became interested in multiprofessional education and research, in which she has been involved for several years. Her MPhil research was comparing and contrasting palliative care in the wider Europe with particular emphasis on the interpretation of the ethos underpinning the specialty. She teaches ethics in a variety of educational programmes and is currently a member of a European Commission Europe-wide project on ethical issues in palliative care. She is Editor of the *European Journal of Cancer Care*.

The study of ethics and the study and practice of healthcare have not merged much in the past, nevertheless ethical standards are essential to the practice of the health professions. Each professional discipline has its own code of conduct, guidelines for practice and philosophy of care to direct practice within its professional remit. There have been several international declarations of human rights within healthcare to protect patients from unethical practices that might nevertheless be portrayed to them as necessary evils in the course of scientific research and utilitarian principles – the greater good.

Despite the relative lack of moral philosophy and healthcare ethics in the curricula of healthcare professionals, it does not take long for anyone in clinical practice to face their first ethical dilemma about which they are called upon to make a judgement or have a view.

In healthcare, appropriate use of professional power compared with the relative vulnerability of the lay client/patient during a first meeting establishes the relationship for all future transactions and establishes trust between the two parties. In the context of progressive illness there are many occasions which will challenge this relationship as the illness trajectory takes its course. There is an increasing number of situations which pose ethical dilemmas whether it be in the equal allocation of resources, equal accessibility to healthcare services, decisions about the right treatments or best care, and the right to life or to end life. All of these examples raise the ethical principles of justice, or fairness, autonomy, beneficence and non-maleficence.

Some health carers may have studied moral philosophy as part of their general education or pursued it as a personal interest. Others may have no grounding at all in this subject. In either case applying moral philosophy to the real world of work with patients in health services, driven by political agendas, is difficult.

Justice for all is an easy phrase to use, but how does one decide whether either a young woman with breast cancer whose only apparent chance of survival (and possibly cure) is an expensive course of drugs or a young child with cystic fibrosis whose only chance of survival is a heart-lung transplant should be allocated the resources from a finite pot where there is money for only one of these two? How can provision be made to satisfy a palliative care patient's autonomy to remain in their own home, when the only way to achieve that is to enlist the support of a reluctant and uncooperative relative to act as the main carer and again, to find the financial resources for professional backup and support?

Professional education and training

Apart from the knowledge-base of moral philosophy, the most important function of studying ethics is to encourage logical, reasoned thinking rather than an unreasoned knee-jerk reaction to a given situation in everyday work.

In medical practice the code of medical conduct – the Hippocratic Oath – which used to be sworn by newly qualified doctors was reinforced by the more recent international codes and declarations formulated as a result of disregard for human rights through human experimentation and sometimes, violation.

These codes include the Nuremburg Code and the Geneva Convention in the 1940s, and the Declaration of Helsinki in the 1960s, amended in the 1970s, which was followed by discussion on national codes of ethical medical practice in the United States of America and Europe and the development of the Institute of Human Values in Medicine (USA). Details of all of these can be found in the text and appendices of several publications, the most recent of which is Campbell et al (1997).

The deficit in the teaching of ethics for doctors resulted in the British Medical Association calling for all medical schools to provide substantial medical ethics and human values teaching in 1986 and in the GMC's recommendations that the doctors of tomorrow need to have such education (GMC, 1996). These are now part of the regular medical curricula in several countries, including the USA and the UK.

Other healthcare professionals have their own codes of conduct or guidelines for practice, which include patient rights and professional responsibilities. They too now have some regular input to their first level training and post-registration courses at all levels, for in-depth study of ethics as it applies to healthcare.

However, codes of conduct and guidelines for practice are only part of the story. They give some parameters within which to work, but they do not necessarily guide one's thinking through an ethical dilemma (such as those already quoted above) to encourage formulation of a viewpoint or judgement.

Clinical trials

Much of the debate on ethical issues in healthcare has been related to the inclusion of human subjects in clinical trials primarily for cancer and psychiatry. The majority of ethics committees were established to scrutinise research protocols for these trials. International protocols have to be seen and agreed by the national and local ethics committees before each of the countries involved can sign up to the trial and before the final scan for ethical practice by the relevant pharmaceutical company. In the UK some of the regional and, even more, local ethics committees have extended their roles to consider other kinds of research proposals to ensure appropriate ethical practice, but these are currently in the minority and are by no means available in all regions.

RESEARCH ETHICS

Consideration needs to be given to the ethical issues involved in all the elements of research, not just those for human experimentation. These include choosing the appropriate methods to do the research; the choice of an appropriate sample; the issue of inclusion of patients and/or their relatives; confidentiality for the research subjects; adequate funding and resourcing to complete the work and so on. All are important considerations for the researcher.

PALLIATIVE CARE

What does all of this have to do with the practice of palliative care? Clinical trials have only just begun in this specialty and other research has been slow to develop. Palliative care is still an emerging specialty and is only now adding to the earlier successes of systematic investigation into pain management and the early studies on bereavement. Now a wide range of issues are the subjects of research through the use either of quantitative or qualitative methods or a combination of these.

The reasons given for not establishing an evidence-base for palliative care earlier were sometimes muddled and sometimes realistic. It was considered that any research with the seriously ill or dying was intensely intrusive. There were instances when this would be the case but others where those facing an imminent death would have been pleased to share even that intensely private and lonely experience with those who were keen to learn from it. Systematic investigation of peoples' feelings, symptoms, anxiety levels and life quality are all now included in research topics. Intrusion into a patient's life is still recognised as a potential problem but great care can be taken in the design of the research to counter or minimise this and so give greater compliance from patients.

Attrition rates can pose a greater problem in palliative care compared to other specialties and have to be considered carefully as part of the research design. One way of minimizing the effects of this is to extend the sample size by collaboration between several centres rather than undertaking more parochial and local research projects.

The usual controls for increasing the number of variables balanced with the sample size need to be adhered to. With palliative care services being offered much earlier in the illness trajectory, some of these issues are less problematical than they once were. Patients may live longer than the terminal care patient of late and their illness may be less severe.

Patients have not been the only subject of research. Carers have also played a very significant part in adding to the palliative care knowledge-base, particularly in the areas of loss and bereavement and in the very important aspects of caring.

ETHICS IN PRACTICE

There are many instances in the everyday practice of palliative care rather than the research into it, when decisions have to be made that include ethical, clinical and practical issues. Any or all of the four main ethical principles appropriate to healthcare may need to be considered and debated. The four principles are beneficence, non-maleficence, autonomy and justice.

Ethics is not just a matter of opinion but requires reasoned and rational thinking to arrive at several possible solutions to a dilemma and then to find the most appropriate one in the circumstances, using these four principles as a basis for the reasoning. However, it must be acknowledged that there are different interpretations to the meaning of the four principles. (See also Jeffrey, Chapter 2.)

JUSTICE

For example, in the case of justice, is it just to respect and provide what are seen as a person's rights – in this context, good palliative care services – in the knowledge that, at least in a democracy, a person has the right to medical treatment and healthcare? If so, what if there are only sufficient resources for one person when two require them simultaneously?

Should justice be interpreted as what someone deserves or needs – rather than necessarily his right? In the former case one could easily be trapped into the meritocracy argument. This person has never smoked a cigarette and yet has developed lung cancer. Should he have the best treatment for his cancer rather than the person who has smoked cigarettes all his life? Another example may be to give treatment or allocate resources to someone who is still able to contribute economically to society compared with a physically or mentally disabled person or someone of older age who has less chance of doing so? Is the only contribution to make an economic one? Marginalizing the disabled and the elderly is regrettably common in society generally and is certainly the case in healthcare.

In the issue of needs, should those who have the most perceived needs – the poor, the sick, the socially disadvantaged – receive first, before those who are privileged, despite similar medical requirements?

HARM (MALEFICENCE)

What is the definition and meaning of harm? If the whole ethos of palliative care is to make the very best of the life that is left, then the relative risks and benefits of all proposed treatment and care need to be considered by the patient (with or without their relatives as they wish) and the professional carers. There is frequently considerable disagreement about what constitutes 'harm' for an individual. The disagreement may be between two health professionals. For example, pain is perceived by doctor 'A' as the cause of most harm to patient X, therefore morphine should be given to relieve it despite its sometimes unwanted effects on the central nervous system of initial drowsiness and impaired concentration (which could also be caused by the pain itself). A second doctor, 'B', may consider that whilst pain is present and in their view is causing harm, there are less effective analgesics than morphine but ones that would limit the unwanted effects on the CNS. Pain would be reduced but not eliminated and concentration and alertness would be retained. The partially-relieved pain may itself impair concentration to some extent but not so much as with the effects of morphine. What are the relative benefits and risks to quality of life for such a patient?

Then consider the patient's perspective. He does not perceive his pain as the worst harm. He is a practising lawyer and wants to continue working despite his serious illness. Work is his main *raison d'etre*. He wants to drink alcohol for his pain (which he is well used to doing). For him it partly relieves his pain, makes him relaxed which also helps to reduce the pain and, because of his tolerance to it he retains a sharp, incisive mind to continue his work.

This example causes a problem for the professionals. Whilst alcohol may be taken in moderation, the amounts that this patient is used to would be considered by them as harmful. They know what will do good in reducing the patient's pain but they are torn between their convictions and the need to respect the patient's autonomy.

JUSTICE AND AUTONOMY

The principles of justice and autonomy can cause similar dilemmas. Justice – rights and responsibilities – is often portrayed as 'I' have rights and 'you' have the responsibility to provide for them, rather than the two in balance. Patients' rights have been the subject of much recent discussion, perhaps in an attempt to redress the many years of paternalism which was little short of coercion at times. That having been said, there are positive aspects of paternalism which still sometimes have a place in healthcare.

Whilst in the palliative care setting patients have some moral rights – to fair and equal treatment and care, to privacy and confidentiality, to autonomy and to information and to the truth – they also have some responsibilities.

If a contractual alliance to plan care together is established between patient and professional, then there are responsibilities to fulfil on both sides of the alliance. One could also argue that satisfying a patient's rights may infringe the rights of another patient, a relative, or a health professional. A clear example of this is the current cry of a patient's 'right to die' when they may wish the professional to help them to end their life and therefore run the risk of implicating them in their death. This can be seen as an infringement of the professional's right to properly and legally practice his profession. There is a whole chapter on this particular issue later in this book (Prouse, Chapter 6).

Conclusions

Why is it important to study ethics, particularly in relation to palliative care? Clearly there are ethical issues and dilemmas to be considered every day in palliative care, just as there are clinical ones. The two really are inseparable. The decision to re-hydrate a patient in the last days of life has clinical implications and ethical ones. The decision to retain a seriously ill patient in an inpatient unit for care because there are inadequate support services in their own home to deal with the extent of difficult symptoms (despite their own wish to be at home), poses clinical as well as ethical issues. Each individual human story is complex and often difficult to resolve at all levels. Each situation needs to be considered in a logical, objective way as well as an emotional, human one and then a balanced view needs to be taken.

The study of ethics is important to enable such reasoning to take place in the context of an understanding of the moral issues that are part of all of our practice. Several innovative ways of teaching ethics have been proposed and tried in palliative care. It is well worth looking at these models from the literature. It is also valuable to search for models of teaching ethics in other specialties with a view to replicating them in the care of the seriously ill. Much work has already been successfully achieved.

In addition to the theoretical input to educational programmes on applied moral philosophy, Burman (Chapter 7) has addressed the teaching of ethics in the practice setting for palliative care. There is no doubt that simulating hypothetical examples of frequently occurring ethical dilemmas for use in teaching (particularly multiprofessional teaching) is extremely valuable. Extending these ideas into 'rehearsing' real situations that are likely to occur for individual patients is also helpful. Anticipating potential dilemmas and discussing them with other professional colleagues is helpful planning for the real event when time may well be against one.

The study of ethics is every bit as important as the study of each individual's main professional discipline – medicine, nursing, religion, social work or whatever. In this crucial time in a patient's life, when life itself is limited and under threat (and you have warning of that, compared with sudden death), every opportunity should be taken to reason with them the best path to tread for all concerned. There will never be one right answer to a dilemma, just a series of possible solutions from which to select the best.

References

Campbell A, Charlesworth M, Gillett G, Jones G. (1997). *Medical Ethics*. Auckland: Oxford University Press.

General Medical Council (1996). *Tomorrow's Doctors*. London: GMC.

CHAPTER TWO

Care versus cure

David Jeffrey

Dr David Jeffrey MA FRCP (Edin) is a Macmillan Consultant in Palliative Medicine at the Three Counties Cancer Centre, Gloucestershire and Honorary Senior Lecturer at the Department of Palliative Medicine, Bristol University. He was formerly a general practitioner and educational training course organiser. He is author of *There is nothing more I can do*, an introduction to ethics in palliative care.

A study of the ethical dilemmas encountered in the course of a serious life threatening illness reveals a tension between the concepts of caring and curing. Although palliative care is not limited to any one diagnostic group, it may be helpful to consider the patient with cancer as a paradigm for this ethical analysis. In the next decade, Western society faces the challenge of caring for an increasingly ageing population with limited resources. Deaths from cancer account for 24 per cent of all deaths in such a society. Thus the patient with cancer is an appropriate model to explore issues surrounding caring and curing.

A diagnosis of cancer may be perceived by a patient as a sentence of death. It is not simply a premature death, but the likelihood of an undignified, painful process of dying, which frightens patients with cancer. Once cancer is diagnosed the world becomes unpredictable. People generally have a need to be in control; uncertainty is difficult to bear. Furthermore, in ordinary language 'cancer' is used as a metaphor for evil. As long as cancer continues to be an 'invincible predator' which is 'obscene' and 'repugnant' then it is likely that patients will be devastated by knowledge of their diagnosis (Sontag, 1979).

The care of a patient with cancer may be divided into phases, each determined by the primary aim of treatment: curative, palliative and terminal (Ashby and Stofell, 1991).

Palliative care is defined by the World Health Organization in the following terms:

The active total care of patients whose disease is not responsive to curative treatment. Control of pain, of other symptoms and of psychological, social and spiritual problems is paramount. The goal of palliative care is achievement of the best quality of life for patients and their families.

Many aspects of palliative care are also applicable earlier in the course of the illness in conjunction with anticancer treatment.

Palliative care neither hastens nor postpones death; provides relief from pain and other distressing symptoms; integrates the psychological and spiritual aspects of care, and offers a support system to help the family cope during the patient's illness and in bereavement (WHO, 1990).

THE CURATIVE PHASE

In the curative phase of treatment there is a realistic chance of cure or long lasting remission. The aim of treatment is survival of the patient. Some harmful side effects of treatment may be acceptable to the patient when balanced against a good chance of cure (Ashby and Stofell, 1991).

At the time of Hippocrates, holistic health and cure were thought to result from spiritual wellbeing. The purpose of medicine was not to identify localised lesions but to explain illness in terms of the total mental and physical disposition of the patient. Caring was an integral part of curing. The linking of the term 'cure' to medical treatment developed in the seventeenth century with the advent of the Cartesian revolution. This dualistic philosophy separated the workings of the mind and body, and interpreted cure as the removal of physical disease (Faithfull, 1994). Medicine then became concerned with specific anatomical lesions which could be linked to the symptoms of disease. This narrow concept of cure has tended to focus medical attention on removing physical disease rather than exploring the broader notion of the subjective aspects of illness (Faithfull, 1994).

The introduction of anaesthesia, modern surgery and antibiotics gave doctors a potential to cure disease. The scientific advances of the twentieth century have encouraged oncologists, radiotherapists and cancer surgeons to adopt a biological view of cancer. Cancer is perceived as an organ dysfunction, rather than an illness which affects the whole person. In the quest for the certainty of clinical cure, doctors risk failing to understand the meaning that experiencing cancer has for the patient. The patient's perception of cure is related to his illness, as a return to the normality which existed before the diagnosis, whilst the doctor's is centred on the disease, in terms of five year survival.

Although, historically, cure has not been a concept which patients have associated with cancer, with earlier diagnosis and an advancing medical technology, patients with cancer and their families may now have high expectations of modern medicine's power to cure. Such expectations may be fuelled by media reports of 'breakthroughs' in cancer treatment, by medical optimism or by a cultural fear of death.

Advanced medical technology has given doctors the potential not only to cure certain cancers but also to prolong the process of dying. For instance, the encouraging results of curative treatments in some types of leukaemias have led to the use of chemotherapy regimes for patients with solid tumours such as bowel cancers where results have been disappointing. At first, such technology was applied indiscriminately to extend life even in those cases where the underlying disease was not curable (Brody, 1988). Such practices came to be considered inappropriate by professionals, patients, their families and the public. Thus currently a tension exists between the availability of life-prolonging treatments with significant side-effects and a desire to resist the use of such therapies where the quality of life of the patient cannot be maintained.

Today, many doctors are concerned with applying a sophisticated technology to remove disease: the medical concept of cure. Success tends to be measured in years of survival, not in terms of quality of life or freedom from sequelae of cancer. In treatment of a cancer a 'tumour response' may or may not be translated into a survival advantage or better control of symptoms (Ashby and Stofell, 1991). Iatrogenic side effects and illness implications may linger for months or years after a person experiences cancer treatment which has been medically defined as curative (Loescher et al, 1989). In a study of 20 individuals pronounced cured, researchers found an enduring sense of vulnerability and evidence that reminders of their illness lingered (Shanfield, 1980). Failure of cure in the context of cancer presents particular difficulties for patients facing the unknown and for professionals who feel they may have failed (Hurny, 1994).

The dilemma for a professional is when to continue to strive to prolong a patient's life and when to focus care on the patient's quality of life and cease active therapies: the dilemma of care versus cure (Brody, 1988).

Care may be defined as serious attention and thought – a person taking caution not to damage or lose, protecting, taking charge of and supervision of (Oxford Reference Dictionary, 1986). The earliest use of the word dates back to the twelfth century.

Someone who cared put themselves in a balanced state of mind, providing for the individual, the emotion of sharing with the other their predicament and therefore easing the burden of the person being cared for (Eyles, 1995).

Caring can be caring about somebody or caring for somebody, or it may imply looking after somebody (Brown et al, 1992). It involves the capacity to feel for another person and the capacity to understand something of the situation. In the healthcare context it requires not only an openness to the patient's needs but also a readiness to reflect on the way that professionals make judgments about what it best for the patient. Care is facilitative rather than intrusive and certainly is not invasive (Barker, 1989).

Much of the literature on caring in a health context is based on nursing practice. Doctors have followed the traditional medical model of care, based on a duty of beneficence. This requires the doctor to do his best for the patient and requires that he causes no harm to come to them as a result of his treatment (non-maleficence). A conflict may exist between a doctor's duty of beneficience, to do what is best for his patient, and his duty to respect the patient's autonomy.

Philosophers offer a variety of definitions of autonomy, each focusing on certain facets of this elusive concept. Gillon stresses rationality and liberty in his definition:

Autonomy is the capacity to think, decide and act on the basis of such thought and decision, freely and independently (Gillon, 1985).

In expressing autonomy, an individual shapes and gives meaning to his life. In a situation where death is, or is thought to be, imminent, then respect for the patient's autonomy assumes a particular importance. For example, a doctor who believes that a patient with advanced cancer would benefit from a course of chemotherapy which could extend his life for a few weeks may be tempted not to disclose the poor prognosis to the patient for fear that he might reject the treatment. By withholding this information, the doctor is acting paternalistically.

Paternalism involves the interference of a patient's autonomy which is justified by referring exclusively to the welfare, good, happiness, needs, interests or values of the person being coerced (Dworkin, 1972).

Paternalism is a denial of autonomy and a substitution of an individual's judgments or action for his own good.

It has been argued that a holistic approach to care is a form of paternalism (Girad, 1988). The holistic approach may increase patient expectations and tends to make the patient dependent upon health carers (Girad, 1988). Such arguments ignore a central characteristic of caring which is the sharing of mutual respect for the autonomy of both patient and professionals. Thus caring rejects paternalism and works towards shared realistic goals. The care-giver does not necessarily have any moral advantage over the care-receiver (Daly, 1987). The process of dying can be a period of moral development for both patient and professional. Classical philosophical thinking on virtue offers insights into the essential moral nature of caring. In adopting a caring approach a member of the healthcare team may develop his/her moral awareness and hence their moral character and professional maturity. Professional morality and wisdom are developed in the process of confronting ethical dilemmas. These dilemmas may have no 'right' answer yet demand a decision.

Ethics is not solely concerned with abstract arguments but also with the practicalities of supporting patients who may be distressed. Sharing may involve both doctor and patient acknowledging their own vulnerability and limitations. Such a close moral relationship requires trust, compassion and the involvement of doctor, nurse and patient. Inequalities of power may act to prevent patients from expressing their views. Sharing involves listening to patients. A partnership between doctor, nurse and patient acknowledges the differences in power but also recognises that all individuals have equal moral status.

Palliative care

Generally, doctors and nurses are more comfortable when treating patients when the goal is cure. In palliative care, the aim is to maximise the patient's quality of life. The transition from a curative to a palliative approach may be filled with uncertainty. The doctor or nurse may feel, or even say, 'There is nothing more I can do' (Jeffrey, 1993).

In contrast to curative treatment, emphasis is placed on the caring aspects of the palliative phase. It is the scientific approach to cure which provides a stark contrast to palliative care, where care is concerned as much with the subjective feelings of the patient and the impact of the illness on the social, emotional and spiritual aspects of his life as with the physical disease.

Ashby's risk-benefit analysis model implies that treatment side effects in palliative care should be less harmful than effects of cancer itself (Ashby and Stofell, 1991). Palliative care involves much more than the control of distressing symptoms. It aims to relieve suffering, a more subtle concept which extends to the way in which illness, rather than a disease, affects the whole individual. The term 'palliation' was first used in a medical context in the sixteenth century to describe the alleviation of suffering. Palliative care acknowledges the interrelated distress of patient, family, nurse and doctor (Cherny et al, 1994). For doctors and nurses to deny emotions and feelings of vulnerability in themselves and in their patients is to deny compassion, and to distance themselves from patients (Alderson, 1991). Compassion is an essential part of the nurse-doctor-patient relationship.

In the palliative phase there is a shift in emphasis from quantity of life to quality of life (George and Jennings, 1993). This shift has an important consequence: a requirement to listen to the patient's views. The recognition of the existence of a natural dying process is central to the ethics and practice of palliative care. Here, care is as concerned with the whole person as with the pathology of the disease. Palliative care demands a multidisciplinary approach rather than a medical one. Palliative care is a complex concept. It incorporates a palliative approach to treatment, which is part of good medical practice; and the utilization of palliative treatments, which includes techniques such as defunctioning ostomies, debulking surgery, orthopaedic fixation, paracentesis. Any of these may be applied at earlier stages of the disease without necessarily adopting holistic palliative care.

Specialist palliative care is a body of knowledge, skills and training programmes which defines the activity of particular doctors and nurses. (Thorpe, 1993)

Palliative medicine may be defined as the study and management of patients with active, progressive, far-advanced disease for whom the prognosis is limited and the focus of care is the quality of life. (Doyle, 1993)

The specialty of palliative medicine is thus defined in terms of the stage of disease progress rather than of any particular pathology, body system or technical approach to management (Doyle, 1993). Although, by using the term 'active', conditions such as dementia and stroke are excluded, the term 'progressive' implies the need for an accurate baseline diagnosis. However, this definition seems to exclude those patients who may benefit from short-term referral to palliative care services early in the course of their disease. Cancer is called advanced when in someone's clinical judgment it is no longer reversible (Cassem, 1985).

Palliative care is provided when introduction to or continuation of curative treatment is not possible or is inappropriate (Sutherland et al, 1993). Palliative care thus may include curative treatment of secondary conditions where this improves quality of life. Similarly, palliative therapies may be appropriate at an early stage of the disease, when the main aim of treatment is cure. It seems illogical to leave patients in pain or distress whilst they are receiving active anticancer therapy, and only deal with these symptoms at a later stage when they are recognised as 'palliative' (MacDonald, 1995). Any distressing symptom ignored early in the illness trajectory may be more difficult to control in the last stages of the illness.

It appears that there is a difference between palliative care and palliative medicine (Pennell and Skevington, 1994). This perhaps reflects a perception that medicine is the art or science of the prevention or cure of disease. It involves an active 'doing' based on scientific knowledge. Care is offering professional solicitude for another person and implies a more passive 'being' process. Caring acknowledges patients' suffering, legitimises the experience and gives people a feeling of personal integrity and value (Suchman and Matthews, 1988). The fact that both these terms are used within palliative care suggests the existence of uncertainty about the basic concept of palliative care within the discipline itself. If those who work in the specialty have difficulty in identifying the underpinning philosophy, how much harder it must be for those outside the profession (Pennell and Skevington, 1994).

Much of the philosophy and knowledge of palliative care was developed within the hospice movement. Hospice care is flexible, individualised, supportive care including palliative care when appropriate, provided in a hospice or elsewhere, which aims to achieve the best quality of life for the patient and family and continues into bereavement for as long as necessary (Sutherland et al, 1993). The establishment of hospice care represents a compromise between the over-enthusiastic application of technology to prolong life and the realization that most dying people do not wish to endure the personal indignities these technologies may involve (Charlton et al, 1995).

The greatest confusion appears to relate not so much to the need for palliation but to the timing of it in the spectrum of care (Doyle, 1993). An acceptable definition is needed for several reasons. There may be resentment from other specialists that palliative care specialists are taking over when all that is needed is the palliative approach. In addition, general practitioners need a clear idea of what exactly is being offered to their patients by palliative care specialists. Patients and their families also need to know what the term means so that they have a clear idea of the goals of care and the resources available to support them (Roy and Rapin, 1994). If the patient seems to be resisting attempts at cure, a clear concept of palliative care may give the professional carers permission to address these issues while curative treatment is still being attempted (Pennell and Skevington, 1994). In attempting to acknowledge the patient as a person first, the palliative care worker is exposed to the stresses of resolving ethical dilemmas and dealing with his/her own pain and grief. A smooth transition between curative, palliative and terminal phases of care is facilitated by facing the issues of death and dying. Death denying attitudes with unrealistic expectations of medicine from both patients and doctors are sources of distress for patients with incurable cancer (Ashby and Stofell, 1991).

THE TRANSITION FROM CURE TO PALLIATIVE CARE

In the cancer context, clinicians offer differing definitions of the starting point of palliative care. Calman states that palliative care begins when the diagnosis of cancer is established, death is certain and likely in the near future, and a curative approach to care has been abandoned (Calman, 1988). This statement does not help us in deciding when to abandon a curative approach. It also seems to exclude situations where 'aggressive' chemotherapy is given with apparent curative intent to patients with widespread cancer who would more reasonably be seen as palliative care patients.

Predicting when death is going to occur may be difficult. Specialist palliative care nurses and hospice units emphasise the importance of early referral of patients, if the highest standards of care are to be achieved. On the other hand, general practitioners are often faced with uncertainty about the rate of progress of the disease and defer referral to such specialists until 'the end'.

It is often difficult to know when to switch to palliative care. It may be hard for doctors to acknowledge that they are not able do any more to cure and they may have feelings of anxiety and guilt.

Although at a rational level a situation may be clearly palliative, the patient and physician may unconsciously push a goal approaching 'cure' rather than acknowledge palliation. It is also possible that the reverse may occur. For example, when patients with some forms of metastatic cancer are not treated, when prolonged remission may be achievable if they were (Hurny, 1994). A tension exists between a tendency to 'overtreat' and 'overinvestigate' and a fear of 'neglecting' the patient (Kearsley, 1989).

Honest communication is essential if patients, their families and doctors are to share common aims of treatment. If there has been · deception from the start, then doctors will find it more difficult to inform the patient that a cure is no longer possible. Relatives who have drawn doctors into colluding with them to deceive the patient may exert pressures to continue inappropriate treatment aimed at cure. Inappropriate treatments may cause harm in a number of ways. Physical suffering may result from the side effects of such treatment, for example hair loss and vomiting from chemotherapy. Distress may also be caused by raising false hopes in the patient and family. Such inappropriate treatment encourages patients, relatives and doctors to avoid the reality of death. Instead, time should be spent helping the patient to come to terms with death and to complete unfinished business. On a wider scale, the inappropriate use of expensive treatments is wasteful of limited medical resources which might have been used to benefit other patients (Rees, 1991).

Chemotherapy is often given with palliative intent; it is therefore important to assess the effect of chemotherapy on quality of life, and whether it actually does relieve symptoms, that is, has a palliative effect. There is a widespread tendency to underestimate the toxicity of treatment (Kearsley, 1986), which returns one to the previous argument of risk versus benefit. Chemotherapy is sometimes used as a way of offering hope in an otherwise apparently desperate situation

(Brett, 1988). But, since this form of treatment carries such a risk of toxicity and does little to meet patients' real needs for honest, sensitive communication, it should not be used to give false hope.

DECISION MAKING AT THE BOUNDARIES OF PALLIATIVE CARE

We need to have a clearer understanding of which treatments are curative, palliative or experimental in each clinical setting (Ashby and Stofell, 1991). George and Jennings suggest that clinical decision making is more difficult when it is certain that the patient will die despite our best efforts (George and Jennings, 1993). However, it may be that greater uncertainty exists at an earlier stage of disease, when clinicians may be caught in a dilemma between over-treating patients on the one hand, or neglecting some remote chance of cure on the other.

In palliative care, health may be perceived as an ability to conclude life appropriately and to get meaning out of that living until death (Pennell and Skevington, 1994). Patients may be suffering an unresolved past, an unsatisfactory present and a lost future. There is often this blurring between acute treatment and palliative care. George and Jennings suggest that we have to become problem-solving and perspective-solving with respect to our patient (George and Jennings, 1993). We have to balance buying time with buying quality. The legitimacy of buying time may be reasonable. There is a need to explain the costs of going down the curative route, in terms of: unfinished business, tasks, relationships and personal resolution. Because the boundaries of care are blurred, it may be more appropriate to shift our attention to respect for the patient's autonomy. George makes a distinction between 'acute palliative' and 'palliative palliative' and feels that a way to resolve this particular dilemma is to break down the barriers between cure and palliative care (George, 1991).

The failure of chemotherapy, radiotherapy or surgery to cure advanced cancer may cause palliative care physicians to neglect their use when they may be helpful (MacDonald, 1995). These therapies can often usefully be used for palliation. Conversely, oncologists may feel palliative care is easing a patient into an earlier death than is necessary. Sadly, a state of two solitudes may exist where the two fail to consult each other adequately. Palliative care physicians must be familiar with advances in oncology. There is a need to integrate palliative care at an earlier stage in the disease trajectory. Furthermore there is recent evidence that general practitioners and primary healthcare teams are uneasy and feel a sense of guilt at the quality of care they are providing for patients with incurable cancer at home (Donald, 1995). Difficulties in professional relationships can raise fears among general practitioners that specialists may take over the care of patients (RCGP, 1995). Hospital care, on the other hand, may not provide a suitable environment for the process of dying (MacDonald, 1995).

Slevin has shown that onclogists vary enormously in their choice of treatment for advanced cancers (Slevin et al, 1990). Mackillop also demonstrates that, while the patient, doctor and family may share a common understanding initially, as time passes and the cancer progresses, patients and physicians may develop divergent views on the aims of the therapy. Patients in a palliative setting may well believe that therapy is aimed at disease control rather than symptom control (Mackillop et al, 1988).

Uncertainties at the boundaries of palliative care

It may be appropriate to identify the uncertainties which exist at the boundaries of palliative care and to clarify the issues involved. The uncertainties involve doctors, nurses, patients and their relatives.

UNCERTAINTIES FOR DOCTORS

There is a risk that doctors lose sight of a cancer's potential to cause death. For instance, in widespread metastatic disease there is a dilemma as to what extent resources should be spent hunting for the primary tumour. Estimating the prognosis for an individual patient is notoriously hazardous. How much of this uncertainty should be shared with the patient? Clinical uncertainty is such that there may be a very real possibility of buying good quality time for someone who may appear moribund, either with aggressive interventions or judicious palliative measures. Who should make the decision to switch from curative to palliative care? Palliative care demands a team approach to care. To what extent should the patient be included in decision making? Reaching a moral consensus within a multi-disciplinary team may be difficult.

Nowadays a conflict often exists between technical care and personal care. In the context of modern medicine, time to listen to patients may be perceived as a luxury. Medical training concentrates on clinical competence. There is a danger that compassion may become a redundant value.

Ethical dilemmas form one of the most challenging aspects of medical care. Struggling with questions which have no obvious answers is an essential part of the professional role. In striving to act with integrity, honesty and a sense of moral responsibility we define what lies at the heart of what it means to be a professional.

UNCERTAINTIES FOR NURSES

Nurses are organised in a hierarchy, whereas doctors work in a collegiate system. This can mean that a nurse may be faced with loyalties divided between patient, doctor and manager.

Much of palliative care is nursing care. Traditionally nurses are closer to patients and more aware than doctors of the patients' wider needs. These needs, which may be psychological, social or spiritual, may be of greater significance to the patient than his/her medical problem. Nurses may be placed in a situation where they have to act as an advocate for the patient. Advocacy is a useful mechanism for power sharing within the team, but all too often it is perceived in a negative way, as a threat, or as implied criticism of medical care. Doctors need to listen to their nursing colleagues who often have a broader view of the patient's concerns.

Nurses may also feel uncertain if there is no clear team philosophy. A patient with advanced cancer may ask a nurse how serious his condition is. How is the nurse to respond if she knows that the consultant always gives an unrealistic optimistic prognosis?

UNCERTAINTIES FOR PATIENTS

Calman defines quality of life in terms of the gap between a person's expectations and the reality of his situation (Calman, 1984). Where there is a wide discrepancy between expectation and reality, then quality of life is low. Calman's model serves to emphasise that part of a doctor's role may be to help patients to have more realistic expectations, particularly at the point where the focus of care is changing from curative to palliative.

Palliative care aims to maximise patient autonomy, so long as it does not adversely affect the autonomy of others (Jeffrey, 1993). Taking responsibility for his choices may mean that the patient will blame himself if events turn out badly. At the interface between curative and palliative care it is particularly important to give patients their final opportunity to exercise their autonomy. Patients are tougher than we think. Part of the task facing the professional carers wishing to give appropriate care is to make some evaluation of the quality of the patient's life. It is important to remember that the most reliable assessor is the patient himself.

Quality of life relates both to objective features of disease and to subjective feelings. The concept of quality of life extends beyond a balance between the impact of a treatment and its side effects to recognise and respect the autonomous individual – the patient – in the social context of his relationships with family and friends.

Patients need just as much information to make rational decisions about their medical condition as they do for any other sphere of their lives. If the doctor is uncertain at the transition of curative to palliative care, he needs to acknowledge his vulnerability and seek to share his concerns with his team, which includes the patient.

UNCERTAINTIES FOR RELATIVES

There may be a feeling of helplessness and a perception that their loved one is suffering. Relatives often fear the harm of giving honest information to the patient. They may insist that the doctor must not tell the patient that cure is no longer possible: 'The news would kill him, doctor'. This is how collusion is born. It develops to isolate the patient from his loved ones, his doctor and nursing staff.

Respect for the patient's autonomy demands that at least he should be the first to know what is happening. This may be difficult if the patient is still drowsy following surgery or when cerebral function is decreased or compromised for some other reason. Professionals can help by suggesting that relatives are present at these discussions.

The relatives may insist that 'something must be done'. Doctors need to explain that palliative care does not mean giving up care. Relatives are often unfamiliar with the features of the normal dying process.

Palliative to terminal care

When in the terminal phase of illness, all unnecessary treatments are withdrawn and 'no treatment-related side effects are acceptable' (Ashby and Stofell, 1991).

The phase of terminal care involves the last days of someone's life, when death with dignity is the aim of care. Relatives may express their distress in terms like 'I would not let a dog suffer like this'. This may surprise the professional carers who see a patient who seems to them, to be dying peacefully. Carers may also become distressed if dying seems to be prolonged. Perhaps patients die as they have lived: some with quiet acceptance, others 'raging at the dying of the light'.

We have a duty of care to ease suffering but not to hasten or prolong the process of dying. In the past, people used to die at home in familiar surroundings, but now there is an increasing trend towards death in hospitals. Dying with dignity means different things to different people. We need to distinguish between euthanasia, control of pain and withholding or withdrawing life-prolonging treatments. Euthanasia is the deliberate termination of someone's life. The control of pain has nothing to do with euthanasia since its purpose is to relieve pain, not to end a life. Withdrawal of treatment in the course of illness occurs when the time arrives when it is no longer possible to restore health, functions or consciousness. It is no longer possible to reverse the dying process. At this stage, the most that even the most aggressive therapy can achieve is to prolong the dying process.

Patients are not obliged to undergo treatment that is futile, and physicians are not obliged to begin or to continue such treatments. Doctors need to accept that death is a part of life; death may come as a relief, but it is not an option for doctors as means of achieving relief (George and Jennings, 1993).

Doctors may, however, be placed in a difficult situation by relatives who equate continuing active treatment with maintaining the patient's hope and morale (Faithfull, 1994). These attitudes are one consequence of the medicalization of death. Death is no longer a familiar natural event and dying is often perceived to be a frightening, painful process which should occur in hospital, where those who know about it can manage it properly.

MULTIDISCIPLINARY TEAMWORK

Patients with cancer present a wide range of physical and emotional problems which can threaten to overwhelm the individual doctor or nurse. A team of professional carers from differing disciplines who share the aims of palliative care, can have the strength and skills to meet the various needs of the patient. However, working in multidisciplinary teams can lead to interprofessional rivalries, leadership difficulties, delayed decision making and may generate unrealistic patient expectations (Fottrell, 1990). Thus ethical problems of interprofessional power sharing can have a detrimental effect on patient care.

Successive NHS reorganizations have not made multidisciplinary working any easier. However, professionals do need to define their areas of expertise so that each understands the other's potential contribution to care. Specialist nurses whose skills are not recognised may become demoralised and deskilled if they are not allowed to make an appropriate contribution. No individual member of the team should be seen as less significant than another.

As professionals, we need to acknowledge the moral challenge of seeing the patient as a whole person by sharing access to the patient. The sad alternative is to witness the prospect of doctors and nurses taking care to maintain their interprofessional boundaries, to the detriment of the patient and her family. Respecting the autonomy of fellow professionals in different disciplines breaks down inter-professional boundaries and creates a team spirit directed to achieving the aims of palliative care.

The vital 'care' component of nursing work is difficult to identify and measure. It is this 'caring' element which is vulnerable to an organization driven by economy and efficiency. Such market forces operating within the NHS have threatened the provision of the 'invisible' components of the holistic care of dying patients (Field, 1989). Nurses want to work as part of a team supporting each other and accepting individual responsibility for their decisions. If doctors and nurse managers do not respect the autonomy of nurses then these nurses will be unable to offer the highest standards of care to their patients. Sharing information within a team is a mechanism for sharing power and for respecting the autonomy of other team members.

If members of a team respect the autonomy of the patient and of fellow professionals then they need to share power and to be willing to accept responsibility for their own decisions. To develop such a sharing relationship is to form a partnership, not just between professional carers but to include the patient.

General practitioners, district nurses, hospital consultants, ward sisters and other healthcare professionals are equal partners and need to recognise each other's skills and roles if they are to meet the needs of patients. Professionals from different disciplines need to communicate and negotiate the optimal plan of care with the patient and her family. This partnership preserves respect for autonomy of both patients and professionals by a process of joint decision making and goal setting (Wilson-Barnett, 1989). Partnership depends upon trust and an acceptance of the patient's view as valid and important. In an every day work situation such trust involves a recognition of the uncertain nature of palliative care in the community. Trust involves supporting the intuitive clinical skills of the team, skills which can only flourish in a secure, safe environment. Expectations of other team members should be realistic and their contribution needs to be acknowledged. A trusting environment allows for open, honest discussion of views which promotes further mutual trust. This type of partnership, underpinned by the ethical principles of respect for autonomy challenges paternalism or individualised leadership by the doctor. It seems illogical to treat patients as equals yet to treat one's colleagues as inferiors merely because they may work in another discipline or may be employees.

MODELS OF CARE

Ethical frameworks based purely on abstract theories of deontology or utilitarianism may seem hard to apply in a clinical situation. Utilitarianism may seem to discriminate against the individual cancer patient whilst the impersonal duties of deontological theory may not be appropriate for the emotional aspects of the care of a patient who is suffering. Both these theories place great weight in pure reasoning and seem to reject and mistrust emotions. They also seem to ignore the practical effects of the difference in power between professionals and their patients.

Similarly, models based on the quartet of autonomy, beneficience, non-maleficence and justice are most useful in abstract analysis but less helpful in the setting of close relationships (Gillon, 1985; Beauchamp and Childress, 1983). If an ethical framework is to be of practical use to patients and staff, respect for autonomy needs to be combined with a caring approach. Such a model has the advantage of acknowledging that feelings, compassions, integrity and virtue play a vital part in the holistic approach to care.

Ethical decisions need to be considered in the context of an individual clinical case and not only in abstract isolation. It is the doctor, rather than the nurse, who makes the decision to change from a curative to a palliative approach. This decision legitimises the patient's entry into the dying process (Field, 1989). Field distinguishes 'clinical death', the absence of life signs such as respiration and heartbeat, and 'social death', which is the process whereby staff, relatives and friends withdraw from the terminally ill. Open honest communication between staff and patients creates a relaxed atmosphere. In this setting, the mutual respect, trust and friendliness between doctors and nurses can lead to their skills being used in an optimal way (Field, 1989). (See also chapters 3 and 5.)

A patient oriented approach concentrates on the need for full information and sets limits on the doctor's perception and beliefs. In his willingness to inform, a doctor reveals his respect for the patient's autonomy.

The central function of informed consent is to ensure a sharing of power and knowledge between doctor and patient. Through this sharing process patients receive appropriate care from doctors they trust, and doctors gain a deeper understanding of the patients' needs.

Informed consent can be viewed as an expression of two elements of care: one responsive to the patient's wishes and the other protective from harmful intervention (Baum et al, 1989). Informed consent is a dialogue between a patient and his doctor in which both become aware of potential harms and benefits for the patient. Informed consent is thus much more than a granting of permission.

There is a need for a better understanding of decision making under conditions of uncertainty at the boundaries of palliative care. Doctors may have a notion of what it is to be 'scientific'; namely, that if the causes of an illness are unclear then more tests must be performed. A conflict exists between this objective attitude and an empathetic approach. We need a model of decision making which combines a requirement for scientific rigour and technical competence with an ethical duty of compassion and respect for the patient's autonomy. We need objective scientific knowledge, but we also need wisdom.

For doctors and patients to face uncertainty together there has to be trust between them. Wise decisions cannot easily be reached in a climate of uncertainty.

Acknowledgment of uncertainty removes a barrier to trust, gives a sense of control over the outcome and offers doctors and patients a chance to be allies not adversaries. Thus by giving up the illusion of total certainty and sharing the reality of uncertainty, we can make more realistic decisions. It is only when we face the fact that we are taking chances that we can begin to make choices. If patients and families are also involved, the doctors gain the benefit of their knowledge and support that comes from sharing the diagnostic and therapeutic dilemmas which previously the doctor has borne alone. Thus more flexible decision making strategies, together with a consideration of a wider range of possible causes, lead to better decisions and better care, and increased trust between doctor and patient.

Our minds get used to thinking in terms of whatever tools we use. If you only have a hammer then every problem looks like a nail. Scientific decision making in curative care can be contrasted with a consensus team approach involving the patient in palliative and terminal care.

George and Jennings have devised a model of decision making based on respect for patient autonomy (George and Jennings, 1993).

Applying a therapeutic index or balancing cost benefit may be expressed visually as a beam, balancing curative (pathology based) and palliative (symptom based) options on a fulcrum of the patient's agenda.

CURATIVE	PATIENT AGENDA	PALLIATIVE
(Pathology Based)	△	*(Symptom Based)*
DIAGNOSIS	TASKS	WASTED TIME
CURABILITY	RELATIONSHIPS	SIDE EFFECTS
PROGNOSIS	UNFINISHED BUSINESS	COMPLICATIONS
BUYING TIME	POLYPHARMACY	BUYING QUALITY

Patients need time for doctors and nurses to listen to their views. Treatment of cancer may have ceased but care of the patient carries on until the moment of death. Society needs to reach an agreement on the proper care of the dying. It is possible that many individuals would be able to die at home with their families, without the use of expensive 'high' technology if they were well informed and allowed choice.

A Caring Model (Jeffrey, 1993)

A partnership between doctors, other healthcare professionals and the patient based on trust and an open honest approach.

- A commitment to teamwork, a partnership between health carers.
- A holistic approach to care.
- Acknowledging uncertainty and vulnerability.

- Listening to the patient.

- Avoiding distancing, sharing emotional involvement and compassion with the patient and her family.

Promoting acceptance of death and resolving unfinished business

- Demystifying cancer and death.

- Acknowledging the value of life and rejecting active euthanasia.

- Accepting that 'letting die' may be permissible in some circumstances.

- Making an appropriate transition between a curative and a palliative approach to care, with the patient's consent and comprehension.

- Taking account of the patient's view of the quality of her life.

Caring for the carers

- Supporting the patient's family.

- Supporting doctors and nurses.

The key to coping with the various uncertainties which arise in beginning and ending palliative care lies in the process of sharing. Doctors need to share their uncertainty with patients and families and with their nursing colleagues. Informed consent is a mechanism for sharing the power of doctors and the patient.

Rapid advances in cancer treatments and the search for cures have created a division between scientific technical care and personalised palliative care. These differing approaches have evolved their own philosophies of care, resulting in the creation of a boundary between curative and palliative care. Palliative care has changed over the past thirty years to become a more scientifically rigorous discipline.

Perhaps it is now appropriate for those adopting technological curative strategies to assimilate some of the holistic approaches of palliative care.

If healthcare professionals work together with the patient in a true partnership of care, respecting his autonomy and seeking his informed and understood consent, then we shall have a better chance of achieving our therapeutic aims, no matter whether they are curative or palliative.

References

Alderson P. (1991). Abstract bio-ethics ignore human emotions. *Bull Med Eth,* May, pp. 13-21.

Ashby M, Stofell B. (1991). Therapeutic ratio and defined phases: proposal of an ethical framework for palliative care. *BMJ*, 302, pp. 1322-44.

Beauchamp TL, Childress JE. (1983). *Principles of Biomedical Ethics.* Oxford: Oxford University Press.

Barker P. (1989). Reflections on the Philosophy of Caring in Mental Health. *Int J Nurs Stud,* 26, p. 135.

Baum M, Zilkha K, Houghton J. (1989). Ethics of clinical research: lessons for the future. *BMJ*, 299, pp. 251-3.

Brett AS. (1988). The patient's expectations in the United States. In: Stoll, B.A. (Ed). *Cost versus Benefit in Cancer Care.* London: Macmillan, pp. 39-49.

Brody B. (1988). *Life and Death Decision Making.* New York: Oxford University Press.

Brown JM, Kitson AL, McKnight TJ. (1992). *Challenges in Caring.* London: Chapman Hall, p. 31.

Calman K. (1984). Quality of life in cancer patients: An hypothesis. *Journal of Medical Ethics*, 10, pp. 124-7.

Calman K. (1988). Ethical implications of terminal care. In: Freeman, M. (Ed). *Medicine, Ethics and Law.* London: Stevens & Sons Ltd., p. 103.

Cassem EH. (1985). Appropriate treatment limits in advanced cancer. In: Billup, J.A (Ed). *Outpatient management of advanced cancer.* Philadelphia: Lippincott & Co., p. 13.

Charlton R, Dovey S, Mizushima Y, Ford E. (1995). Attitudes to death and dying in the UK, New Zealand and Japan. *J Palliat Care*, 11, pp. 42-7.

Cherny NI, Coyle C, Foley KM. (1994). Suffering in the advanced cancer patient: a definition and taxonomy. *J Palliat Care*, 10, pp. 57-70.

Daly ME. (1987). Towards a phenomenology of caregiving: growth in the caregiver is a vital component. *J Med Ethics*, 13, pp. 34-9.

Donald AG. (1995). Palliative care in the community: difficulties and dilemmas. *Proc R Coll Physicians*, 1995, 25: 550-7.

Doyle D. (1993). *The Oxford Textbook of Palliative Medicine*. Eds Doyle D, Hanks G, MacDonald N. Oxford 1993.

Doyle D. (1993). Palliative medicine: a time for definition? *Palliat Med,* 7, 253-255.

Dworkin G. (1972). Paternalism. *Monist*, 56, 64-84.

Eyles M. (1995). Uncovering the knowledge of care. *British Journal of Theatre Nurses,* Vol. 5, No 9, p. 22.

Faithfull S. (1994). The concept of cure in cancer care. *Eur J Cancer Care*, 3, pp. 12-7.

Field D. (1989). *Nursing the Dying.* Tavistock: Routledge.

Fottrell E. (1990). Multidisciplinary functioning: will it be of use? *British Journal of Hospital Medicine*, 43, p. 253.

George RJD. (1991). Palliation in Aids: where do we draw the line? *Genitourinary Medicine*, 67, pp. 85-6.

George RJD, Jennings AL. (1993). Palliative care. *Postgrad Med J*, 69, pp. 429-49.

Gillon R. (1985). *Philosophical medical ethics*. London: John Wiley.

Girad M. (1988). Technical expertise as an ethical form: towards an ethics of distance. *J Med Ethics.* 14: pp. 25-30.

Hurny C. (1994). Palliative care in high-tech medicine: defining the point of no return. *Support Care Cancer*, 2, pp. 3-4.

Jeffrey D. (1993). *There is nothing more I can do: an introduction to the ethics of palliative care*. Cornwall: Patten Press.

Kearsley JH. (1986). Cytotoxic chemotherapy for common adult malignancies: 'the emperor's new clothes' revisited? *BMJ*, 302, pp. 1-2.

Kearsley JH. (1989). Compromising between quantity and quality of life. In: Stoll, B.A. (Ed). *Ethical Dilemmas in Cancer Care*. London: Macmillan, pp. 39-49.

Loescher L.J et al. (1989). Surviving adult cancers, Part 1: Physiologic effects. *Ann Intern Med*, 111, pp. 411-32

MacDonald N. (1995). The interface between palliative medicine and other palliative care services. *Proc R Coll Physicians Edinb*, 25, pp. 558-68.

Mackillop WJ, Stewart WE, Ginsberg AD, Stewart SS. (1988). Cancer patients' perceptions of their disease and its treatment. *Br J Cancer*, 58, pp. 355-8.

Oxford Reference Dictionary New Illustration (1986). Hawkins (edit). Oxford: Clarendon Press.

Pennell M, Skevington S. (1994). Problems in conceptualising palliative care. In: Ed MacLeod R, Jones C. (Eds). *Teaching Palliative Care: Issues and Implications*. Penzance: Patten Press.

Rees GJ. (1991). Cancer treatment: deciding what we can afford. *BMJ*, 302, pp. 799-800.

Roy DJ, Rapin C. (1994). Regarding euthanasia. *European Journal of Palliative Care,* 1, pp. 57-9.

Royal College of General Practitioners and Cancer Relief Macmillan Fund. Palliative Care Facilitator Project. 1995.

Shanfield S. (1980). On surviving cancer: psychological considerations. *Comparative Psychiatry*, 21, pp. 128-34.

Slevin ML et al. (1990). Attitudes to chemotherapy: comparing the views of patients with cancer with those of doctors, nurses and the general public. *BMJ*, 300, pp. 1458-60.

Sontag S. (1979). *Illness as Metaphor*. London: Penguin.

Suchman A, Matthews D. (1988). What makes the patient-doctor relationship thearapeutic? Exploring the connexial dimension. *Ann Intern Med*, 108, pp. 125-30.

Sutherland R, Hearn J, Baum D, Elston S. (1993). Definitions in paediatric palliative care. *Health Trends*, 25, pp. 148-50.

Thorpe G. (1993). Palliative care comes of age. *Hospital Update*, 2, pp. 435-436.

Wilson-Barnett J. (1989). Limited autonomy and partnership: professional relationships in healthcare. *J Med Ethics*, 15, pp. 12-6.

World Health Organization. (1990). Cancer Pain Relief and Palliative Care. *Technical Report Series* 804, Geneva.

CHAPTER THREE

Giving it straight
the limits of honesty and deception

Heather Draper

Heather Draper PhD is Lecturer in Biomedical Ethics in the
Centre for Biomedical Ethics at Birmingham University's Medical
School. She is Director of Studies for an MSc in Healthcare Ethics
and also teaches ethics to medical students and other healthcare
professionals in the West Midlands region. She is a member of the
ULTRA panel, Vice-Chair of West Midlands MREC, part of the
Advisory Committee to the UK Human Tissue Bank and also sits
on a clinical ethics committee for the Assisted Conception Unit in
Birmingham Women's Hospital Trust. She is an active member of
the UK Forum on Heathcare Ethics and the Law. She writes
broadly in the field of bioethics.

Hearing that you are going to die sooner than you hoped, or hearing that the best that medicine can offer by way of a cure hasn't cured you is, for most people, devastating news. We may take out insurance to cover our premature death, but we do not really expect to need it. A terminal diagnosis is perceived by healthcare workers as one of the worst pieces of bad news to give – save perhaps that of telling a parent that their child is beyond cure. It is the kind of news that alters the course of someone's life and puts to an end, at a stroke, all their hopes for the future and many of their perceptions about themselves (for instance, as independent, or competent, or supporting – rather than supported – members of the family). But this news is, of course, not always what the patient most dreads and nor need it herald unadulterated gloom. For patients weary of a dutiful struggle against a long-standing illness, the opportunity to stop fighting the illness and concentrate on living might be welcome. For others, the news, although undesirable, might come with hitherto unconsidered benefits. Although many of us hope for a sudden and painless death, simply never coming home from work one day can be more devastating for our families than coming to terms with a forthcoming death and making plans together for the future up to and beyond the funeral.

Recently, for a close friend of mine, the terrible and unexpected news that her father only had a few more months to live was turned into a tremendous gift, as she and he were reconciled with each other in a way she had never dreamed possible. Both of them would have been robbed of something very precious if he had not been told that he was dying. Moreover, he was able to die in his own home because he was able to discuss openly and honestly his pain relief and other needs with his carers. My friend was able to suspend her studies and return home to help her mother care for him. His death was distressing for all the family and I am sure that the intensity with which my friend still misses him has been heightened by their total reconciliation, but the experience was, nevertheless, a positive one. This is one case where honesty and the best that palliative care could offer turned the bad news into something positive for everyone concerned.

Equally, we have all heard of cases where the news of a pending and premature death heralds the beginning of unremitting misery, hopelessness and defeat. Everyone has experience of a patient who 'turned their face to the wall' and it is impossible to ensure that every patient, no matter how angry and resentful they – or their family – are, will have a peaceful death. In the case above, my friend readily admits that she would never have predicted that her father's premature death would have been such a positive experience. In many respects, none of us know how we will respond until we have to.

In palliative care, being honest with patients about their prognosis has always been considered a first principle – being referred for palliative care at all generally means that patients have been told their prognosis even if they refuse to believe it. Is honesty in palliative care simply a pragmatic requirement – good palliative care may be frustrated unless the patient is dealt with honestly? Clearly not, for receiving good palliative care is not just a matter of receiving the best that palliative care can offer. It impacts on the quality of life and death, relationships, and present and future interests. The use of the word 'good' in 'good palliative' care (or 'good medicine', or 'good nursing' or 'a good doctor' or 'a good nurse') has two meanings. It is both a technical assessment and a moral judgement because maximum health is one of the 'goods' of life. It is a good from which other goods flow and a means to the end of achieving other goods too. Because good healthcare has a moral as well as a technical component, and because giving and receiving healthcare forms relationships, we are likely to ask the same questions about honesty in a therapeutic relationship as we are in any other. Is it obviously the case that in this relationship 'honesty is the best policy'? Should we always 'tell the truth and shame the devil'? We can all think of circumstances where nothing but harm can be caused by an honest reply but we still hold fast to the belief that honesty is a virtue and deception is to be avoided.

There are several possible responses to this problem. The first is that we should always be honest and that when we are not, we are either being weak of will (or cowardly, even), or we are being overly paternalistic. The second is that deception can indeed be a good thing on occasions and that what we need to do is to determine when these occasions arise. The third is that honesty is a character trait that adapts to circumstances and is not to be interpreted as a statement that one never lies or deceives.

Each of these responses can be explained and justified with reference to the central ethical theories of Kantian deontology, utilitarian consequentialism and virtue ethics, and questions about honesty and deception extend beyond those of giving a terminal prognosis. Overlaying all these problems in the therapeutic relationship is the extent to which the professional is under a greater obligation to be honest to the patient than to others, and whether the duty of care may on occasions require a limited amount of deception – perhaps even a degree of deception that would be unacceptable in nontherapeutic relationships. But before we move on to look at theories and other examples in later sections of this chapter, we need to be certain of what it is we mean when we say that we applaud honesty and deplore deceit. Is honesty the same as always telling the truth? Is deception always achieved through lying? These are important questions, for it is not unusual for people to claim that whilst it is permissible to remain silent, it is impermissible to lie – even though the predicted effect is the same. Likewise, it is commonly asserted that it is one thing to tell the truth, but quite another to tell the whole truth because being 'economical with the truth' is not the same as lying.

Distinctions such as these are controversial, and exploring the potential difference helps to clarify not only the terms we use, but also the importance with which they are bestowed.

Honesty and deception, lying and truth-telling: conceptual differences

Todd and Still (1993) surveyed the strategies and tactics of GPs communicating with their terminally ill patients. We would not be surprised to learn that in 1993, many GPs tried to disclose bad news (as they perceived it) often by allowing the patient to dictate the pace at which understanding was reached. What was surprising was that another strategy was to avoid disclosure using the tactics of evasion, denial, uncertainty, hints and prompts, euphemism and inappropriate reassurance. Here are some of the things that GP 20 said about his (or her) means of avoiding the issue.

'I never tell them what they have got... even if the hospital has told them... I always try to make them see it differently... that they didn't understand it... that it is not terminal, it will clear up... I just don't give it [the terminal diagnosis] away... I always try to avoid answering [the patient's questions]... I always try to find a way out of the answer... or I try to be cheerful and change the conversation... They will ask things like, "doctor, do you think I will benefit from going to hospital?" I say "Yes, you will benefit", even if I do not think that they will... I may tell lies like... "we have got a letter from the hospital that they are hoping that you will be all right in the next month or so, but you need to get over the operation"... [once] I just said that I am sorry that I don't have the full [report of] the investigation from the hospital yet... I didn't tell this woman anything... In fact to get out of it I sent one of my colleagues to go instead of me because I knew that she would put me in a corner...

and that worked because she didn't ask him… I told him I couldn't tell her that she had cancer… I don't think he told her anything, she wouldn't have asked him. But I never saw her again.'

It would be seriously unjust to make inferences from the practice of this GP to the practice of healthcare workers generally. What is interesting about this GP is that he (or she) employed several different means of avoiding honest communication with the patient – particularly evasion. Although there is admission of direct lying, something akin to the truth is also being used either to evade or deceive. Imagine a patient asking 'Do you think I have a chance?' being told 'Well, I sincerely hope so'. It may both be the case that one has this sincere hope, but also that it is very unlikely to be realised. The net effect on the patient, however, is likely to be that they do think that it is realistic to hope. In other words, they are as deceived by the truth as they may have been by the straightforward lie 'Yes, I think that you have a chance'. Of course, we can also reconcile ourselves to our deceptions by crossing our fingers behind our backs as we speak, thinking 'There is always a chance, no matter how slight, it is still a chance'. We know that we are deceiving, but we feel better about it because we have not lied.

Examples such as this suggest that the real principle at issue here is not truth-telling but honesty. In medicine, only one thing seems certain and that is that our 'knowledge' of 'the truth' is constantly changing. It is not unlikely that most of what we now believe to be the truth will, in the future, be shown to be mistaken belief. In this sense, we may rarely be imparting 'the truth', however well intentioned and committed to honesty we are. We would, however, draw a distinction between mistakenly misleading someone (because we are mis-informed) and deceiving someone. It is not truth-telling which is important to us but honesty.

Jennifer Jackson (1991) makes several other useful comments on truth-telling. The first is that, whatever we may claim, we actually lie quite frequently. The examples she gives include signing 'Yours sincerely', or responding 'Very well thank you' when we actually barely know the person we are addressing, or feel dreadful. This behaviour is not quite the same as endorsing so called white lies. Little white lies tend to be characterised by the relatively trivial nature of the deception involved. The untruths we tell almost as a matter of protocol or etiquette are different in the sense that they are not meant to be believed. They fall outside the parameters of honesty because we all know the rules. We are not deceived and nor is there any intention to deceive. This leads to a second observation that to deceive, the deceiver has to be believed. I might tell you the most terrible lie, but if you do not believe me, you are not deceived.

There is a difference between the intention to deceive and the success of that intention. It is not obvious that the failure neutralises the act. Whilst it may be consequentially better for intentional deception to fail, there is something morally suspect about this intention which exists independently of the outcome. Jackson's third observation is that people deceive without the intention to do so, for example, because they do not realise the interpretation which has been placed upon their behaviour. However, should they become aware of this deception and fail to correct it, they become party to the deception. It becomes voluntary even though it was not intended. For instance, Nurse Roberts raises his eyebrows to acknowledge the discreet arrival at Ms Ghupta's bedside of a colleague who is late for the ward round. Roberts' gesture coincides with the consultant informing Ms Ghupta that the effects of chemotherapy really are not so bad. Ms Ghupta notices Nurse Roberts' gesture and thinks that it signifies that he disagrees with the consultant's opinion about the chemotherapy. She decides not to consent to the chemotherapy without a second opinion. Nurse Roberts, when talking to her about her decision, realises what has happened, but does not inform Ms Ghupta of her error. Although his original gesture was not intended to misinform Ms Ghupta, he becomes party to her deception when he fails to correct her false impression.

To summarise, it is never possible to be certain that one is telling the truth because one might be misinformed. One can, however, be honest and genuinely misinformed and this suggests that what counts is not the imparting of the truth per se, but the intention to be truthful. It is also possible to deceive someone unintentionally. If, however, this unintentional deception is deliberately left unchecked, then one might be considered to have voluntarily deceived, even though there was no original intention to deceive. Likewise one can intentionally deceive by deliberately manipulating the truth to misinform. This also suggests that it is honesty rather than truth-telling as such which is important. Similarly, deception requires the person on the receiving end to be deceived, which suggests that the dishonesty of the person intending to deceive can be evaluated independently of the good or bad consequences which flow from the intention.

Is there an ethical imperative to be honest?

This seems a strange question to ask because it provokes the response that it is obvious that we should be honest. The problem with this answer is that there are occasions when being honest will do only harm and in such cases it seems at least permissible, if not required, to be dishonest. It is probably our reluctance to let go of the general principle of veracity that causes us to 'fudge the truth' on those occasions where dire consequences will follow if we are honest. After all, hard cases make bad laws. But it is also commonly asserted that healthcare ethics depends upon four principles – autonomy, nonmaleficence, beneficence and justice – and that these principles sometimes conflict with each other, generating the hard cases. Looking to the consequences of our actions – as we must to assess their benevolence or maleficence – permits us to be flexible and recognise that while it is generally benevolent to be honest, it is legitimate to be dishonest on occasions.

This approach would be justified by utilitarianism. Honesty is generally the best policy because without it we could not depend upon people to be honest. A wholesale erosion of trust would be a sufficiently weighty negative consequence to outweigh some specific benefit of dishonesty or problem with honesty. When I ask for directions or for the correct time, I assume that the answer given will be honest (even if it turns out to be mistaken or unclear – as so many directions are!). A general adherence to honesty is necessary for trust to exist between members of society – particularly relative strangers. However, in other relationships including those between patients and carers, a more explicit relationship of trust exists. The quality of the care which we experience depends almost as much upon the trust we have in our carers as it does on their skills and competence. Where trust breaks down, so does care. This is a strong utilitarian reason to be honest, but utilitarianism cannot embrace absolute adherence to rules. Where honesty promotes only harm, then we are free to abandon it. However, cases where honesty promotes only harm are rare. Generally we have to make a balance of harms and benefits which might mean that dishonesty does do harm, but not as much – or so we hope – as being honest would. The balance of harms and benefits in healthcare recognises that the trust of patients is fragile and that benefits generated by dishonesty can be quickly outweighed by the harm of losing a trusting relationship. For instance, if we lie to a patient at the request of a relative we have to consider not only whether a breakdown of trust with the patient will result (should the lie be discovered) but also whether our willingness to lie will jeopardise future relationships which the relative might form with other practitioners. If one practitioner is willing to lie at the request of a relative, how can that relative be certain that another practitioner will not lie to them if requested to do so? We should also consider that even when the predicted good consequences do flow from lying, the deception always harms people to some extent because it undermines their autonomy.

Utilitarianism does give weight to the effect which lying has on autonomy. Mill, for instance, argued that maintaining autonomy itself had vitally good consequences which should never be taken lightly. In this respect, the principles of nonmaleficence and beneficence conflict with the principle of autonomy less frequently than arguments in favour of paternalism often suppose. Doing well for people includes promoting their autonomy, and nonmaleficence can concern itself with the protection of autonomy.

Kantian ethics give a different weight to autonomy than does utilitarianism. Mill's argument for permitting maximum liberty was that a society in which the liberty to challenge the status quo is limited is liable to stagnate and crumble, which is in no one's interests. Kant held that autonomy is inextricably linked to morality and that it was therefore nonsense to be both in favour of morality and willing to undermine autonomy. He argued that it is our capacity to be autonomous which generates ethical duties. This is because to be responsible at all we must be capable of exercising our own will, choosing our own ends, and choosing between courses of action (maxims) which will meet these ends. Kant's second formulation of the categorical imperative (test for moral conduct) was that we should respect the autonomy of others by never using autonomous people solely as a means to our own ends but always treating them as ends in themselves. Being dishonest with someone is an example of treating them as a means to our own ends. For instance, if we lead a patient falsely to believe that his diagnosis is not terminal because we believe that the bliss of ignorance is better than the pain of knowledge, we deprive him of the opportunity to decide for himself which is of greater value. In addition, we deprive him of other choices which he would be in a position to make if he knew the truth about his condition. In both these senses, we make him a means to our ends and we fail to respect his autonomy, depriving him though his ignorance of choice because we prevent him from making critical decisions as a direct result of our deception.

In addition, Kant argued that moral choices were also wholly rational choices and that just as rationality was universal, so too was morality. In this respect his first formulation of the categorical imperative, universality (that we should ask how it would be if everyone did what we were proposing to do), also acknowledges the relationship between honesty and trust. If everyone lied all the time (i.e. if lying were universal) the whole purpose of lying would be undermined because no one would ever believe that they were hearing the truth. Accordingly, it is self-defeating to lie, and irrational to act in a self-defeating way.

Kant furnishes us with two reasons to make honesty an absolute rule. His views about the unconditional value of morality and autonomy enable him to assert that telling lies is always wrong because if something is unconditional – without conditions – it admits no exceptions. It is universal. Interestingly, it is at this juncture that Jennifer Jackson defends the distinction between telling lies and intentional deception. She proposes that whilst lying is always wrong (for the reasons generally attributed to Kant – namely that it is imperative to have an absolute prohibition on lying to maintain trust and autonomy) intentional deception may be benign, and permissible, therefore, in circumstances where it would be wrong to lie. Bakhurst

(1992) disagrees. He argues that since intentional deception and lying amount to the same thing (the patient is denied access to the truth), if lying is wrong (for the reasons given by Jackson) then intentional deception must be equally wrong. Jackson's response to this claim is to draw a distinction between those cases where intentional deception undermines trust (as lying always does) and those cases where it does not (Jackson, 1993). For instance, both intentionally deceiving a patient or lying to her in order to gain her consent to some treatment are equally wrong. One cannot be absolved of the wrongs of lying by substituting intentional deception because, in both cases, the trust which the patient has is undermined (to their detriment in terms of autonomy). Jackson claims, however, that a betrayal of trust 'can only occur in those cases where those being deceived can reasonably have expected not to be' and what we can reasonably expect is culturally determined, not absolute. While she concedes that the present culture of western medicine is autonomy centred, she recognises that it need not be so. It could, for instance, be driven by an understanding of nonmaleficence which is not founded in respect for autonomy. Likewise, by extension, it is possible to envisage that even within our autonomy-centred culture, individual patients might want to base their relationship of trust with their carer, not on the promotion of their autonomy, but on the belief that the carer will always act in their best interests as perceived by the carer ('You decide doctor, I know that you will do what you think is best'). This is a similar, but not identical situation to the one where patients autonomously let their doctors make the decisions ('You decide, doctor, you're the expert').

If this distinction is valid, it removes one of the stumbling blocks to deception in healthcare, palliative or otherwise, namely that patients need to be told the truth in order to consent to therapy. In a model of healthcare where autonomy is the prominent value, consent is vital as an expression of autonomy, and being informed vital to consent. However, we need to remember that this is not the only model of healthcare in operation, and that it is as paternalistic to force a patient to conform to this paradigm as it is to prevent them from doing so if they wish.

This is, however, an extremely limited defence of deception, and one where dishonesty is related only to the betrayal of a particular kind of trust. It is far more common for defences of dishonesty to be made on the basis that autonomy, while important, is not absolutely important and can be outweighed by other considerations – such as different harms to self (e.g. longevity and wellbeing) or the erosion of the autonomy of others or the avoiding of different harms to them. These distinctions, and their significance, are best illustrated with reference to the examples which will be discussed in the following section.

The final theory against which to measure the imperative to be honest is virtue theory. Virtue theory has its origins in ancient Greek philosophy, one aim of which was to discover which kind of life is best for humans to live. It was recognised that what counts as a virtue cannot be determined solely by asking questions about what good is or means because any definition of good is influenced and conditioned by circumstance. For this reason, virtue theory holds that people need to be trained to be good so that they acquire the habit of goodness through practising being good. To be truly virtuous is to know spontaneously what should be done because of the kind of person one is. For this reason, whereas both utilitarianism and Kantian ethics start with the question, 'What should I do?' virtue theory asks, 'What kind of person should I be?'. If I want to be a good palliative care practitioner, I need to know what qualities good palliative care practitioners have. To learn this, I may look around for a role model to emulate, and through emulating this role model, I will acquire virtuous characteristics myself. Virtuous qualities need not be universal – for instance, a good jazz musician will need different qualities to those required for palliative care – but it is likely that some virtues will be common to similar professions.

One criticism of virtue theory is that we need to be able to recognise good practice in order to emulate it, and that we therefore run the risk of perpetuating bad practice. This was the charge levelled against healthcare practitioners some thirty years ago before it was decided – partly due to public pressure and partly due to legal judgements – that practitioners should be encouraged to develop their own skills of ethical judgement. Virtue theory has, however, been growing in popularity in recent years as the professions have begun to return to the view that being a good practitioner owes a great deal to attitude.

The virtue theory view of honesty enables practitioners to be more responsive to circumstances than deontology allows, without binding them to consider only the consequences of their actions, as utilitarianism does. Possessing the virtue of honesty does not commit us to telling the truth on each and every occasion. The virtuous person knows when it is important to be honest and when to exercise discretion. The mark of the virtuous person is that, whatever they do on any one particular occasion, they retain our respect as honourable and upright people, whose judgement is trusted.

Honesty applied

BEING SELECTIVE WITH THE TRUTH

The advantage of thinking in terms of honesty rather than truth-telling is that we can draw a distinction between bluntness and truthfulness and between honest and dishonest selective truthfulness. Children often fall foul of these distinctions when they are told 'always tell the truth' and then proceed to do so indiscriminately – just as the 'always' suggests they should. Honesty can be legitimately tempered with compassion. It is common practice when communicating with patients to let them dictate the pace at which information is given. Breaking news gradually is not dishonest. The 'whole truth' need not be delivered in an instant provided that one intends to make oneself available to respond honestly to requests for more information.

Likewise, it is not dishonest to keep unsolicited opinions to ourselves. For instance, it is not dishonest to keep to oneself the opinion that a family should visit more often, or stay for less time, or address different issues on their visits. Likewise, it is not dishonest of me not to offer the view that your shirt is awful and your breath smells. Similarly, one should distinguish between offering professional advice and personal advice when asked during the course of one's work for advice about what someone should do. When we do offer unsolicited information we may be motivated by considerations other than honesty. For instance, informing a family that their visits are too long might be part of the duty of care owed to a patient who becomes exhausted or distressed during extended visits. There is a sense in which we are always selective with the truth. The practice only acquires negative connotations when the selectivity is part of a conscious effort to deceive.

CONFIDENTIALITY

Further evidence that we are under no absolute obligation to disclose the truth comes by looking at confidentiality. Being truthful or honest is compatible with not disclosing everything we know when we have a duty to maintain confidentiality. The duty of confidentiality attempts to draw a distinction between that which is known and information that, while known by someone else, we own and have a legitimate right to keep to ourselves. We can be party to information which is not ours and which we cannot therefore disclose. This duty is not, however, an uncontroversial one, particularly when there are concerns that others might be harmed as a result of their ignorance, or when rigid adherence to confidentiality is perceived by relatives as being obstructive or antagonistic.

In recent years, discussions about confidentiality have tended to focus on the dangers of refusing to disclose the positive HIV status of a patient to individuals at risk of infection. But a dilemma about whether or not to disclose confidential information can be generated by far less dramatic concerns (Draper, 1997). In palliative care, carers might be asked not to tell relatives about the seriousness of a patient's symptoms or his decision to minimise intervention. But carers have also been asked not to tell relatives apparently good news too, as the following case illustrates.

CASE

Against all the odds, and despite being referred to a hospice, Collette showed signs of recovering from bowel cancer. After several months, the consultant decided that Collette was no longer terminally ill, though he could not be certain that she would not become ill again in the future. Accordingly, he felt that she no longer needed the extensive support supplied by the hospice, and he discharged her. Collette was very cross about this, partly because she found it difficult to believe that she was actually recovering and partly because she did not want to lose her terminally ill status which had generated rather more attention from her family than she had been accustomed to in the past. The hospice staff were not unsympathetic. They had after all promised Collette that they would not abandon her and would care for her until she died. There was also a widely shared belief among the staff that Collette's family had rather neglected her in the years preceding her diagnosis. Because they did not wish to let Collette down, she was given a radically reduced but honorary status as an out-patient. For instance, she still came on some social events and had her hair set by a hairdresser, who donated some of her spare time to the hospice. It quickly became obvious that Collette's family did not realise that she was no longer thought to be terminally ill. The nurse-manager attempted to talk to Collette about this but was politely and firmly told to mind her own business.

DISCUSSION

Collette's circumstances are obviously not usual, and her success in keeping her new prognosis from her family was aided by the attempts of the staff to negotiate a new relationship with her. Whatever one thinks about the wisdom of the staff's decision to maintain a relationship with Collette, the principal argument in support of honesty – namely that it enables autonomous decision making – applies to Collette's family too. It is not unlikely that if they were in possession of all the facts, the family would reduce the company and help they were prepared to give to Collette. Irrespective of how unreasonable their predicted behaviour might seem to either Collette or the staff, neither should prevent the family from making this decision for themselves. However, the staff are obliged to keep Collette's medical history confidential, despite the fact that what they are keeping from the family on this occasion might be classed as good rather than bad news, and despite their judgement that Collette was being imprudent at best, wrong at worst, not to update her family. Clearly, the staff will feel even more awkward about the situation if any of the family begin to ask direct questions. A further cause for concern is the hairdresser who is volunteering her skills to people who are terminally ill. Unless she is informed that Collette is no longer terminally ill, she is being deceived into parting with her voluntary labour every time she sets Collette's hair.

One point to be made about this case, and others like it – even when there is more at stake, as in the case of an undisclosed HIV risk – is that autonomy is double edged. Being responsible for one's decisions – as Collette is asserting she is – not only gives one the freedom to decide for oneself, it also leaves one open to praise or blame for the decisions one makes.

We have already discussed a distinction between autonomously deciding to let other people make one's therapy decisions, and the sort of relationship which is based on a different kind of trust, namely that the carer just does always have one's best interests at heart. Bobbie Farsides in her chapter in this collection on consent discusses these kinds of decisions at length.

One of the problems with the decisions, like those in Farsides' case of Jean (where Jean deliberately excluded herself from decisions about her care) arises if the patient has requested that he or she should not be reminded of their deterioration. Randell and Downie (1996) discuss the case of one such patient with breast cancer in whom metastases in the cervical spine was discovered. This indicated that the patient should take more rest and wear a neck collar to minimise the risk of quadriplegia. In a case such as this, those charged by the patient with her care have to decide whether to talk to the patient about this further deterioration, or respect her wishes not to discuss anything with her. If they respect her wishes, she may not realise the full significance of their advice to wear a neck collar. Farsides' case of Dillon is similar, in that the patient has chosen to be only partially informed about the unscrupulous practices of drug companies.

'NO GOOD CAN COME OF TELLING THEM THE TRUTH'

There are very few cases when there is nothing to be said in favour of honesty. Usually the erosion of autonomy or the adverse effects of discovery carry some weight, even if they are ultimately thought to be outweighed by the harms that being honest could cause.

CASE

Mrs Stretton was under the care of a palliative care consultant in a general care of the elderly ward when she took an unexpected and acute turn for the worst, and died before her family could be with her. The family, as is common in these circumstances, asked about Mrs Stretton's death, whether she said anything or suffered. In fact Mrs Stretton had become very distressed because she realised that she was dying before she expected to, it had not been possible to keep her pain-free and she had asked where her family was.

In circumstances such as these, it might seem more than permissible to intentionally deceive, or even lie. Telling her family cannot change Mrs Stretton's experience of death, and they could be plunged into guilt and remorse about something over which they had no control.

However, there are occasions similar to these where even though no good can be generated in the particular circumstances, dishonesty might store up trouble in the future. Imagine if Mrs Stretton had not been told that she was terminally ill, at the explicit request of her family. Imagine further that the staff against their better judgement had acceded to these wishes even though they believed that Mrs Stretton's care was compromised, particularly when she realised that death was imminent. Although one might still be tempted to keep the distress of her death to oneself, greater thought would need to be given to reassuring her family that they did the right thing in not telling her she was dying.

We need to draw a distinction in this context between repeatable and unrepeatable occurrences. Clearly, if the event is unrepeatable the assertion that nothing can be gained and only harm can be done looks valid. Since, however, it is likely that the family will have to deal with terminal illness on future occasions, it is highly desirable that they learn from their mistakes – however painful this might be at the time.

Palliative care was one of the first specialities to take team, or shared care seriously. Honesty plays an important role in building a strong team. Everyone must feel able to voice support or misgivings, to acknowledge their mistakes and triumphs, and to take as well as give without fear or resentment.

But teamwork also has its problems. It is not clear where the responsibility lies for decisions made by a team. Is it like a democracy where all agree to accept the decision of the majority, or do individual members have a veto? Does the most senior member of the team carry ultimate responsibility or are all equally and jointly liable for any mistakes which are made? Does one person canvass the opinion of all and form a final judgement based on these views, or does the team have to reach a compromise on which everyone can agree?

Teams that have resolved these and other problems are likely to be well established, with a history of trust and loyalty between members. What would a member of such a team do if she discovered that a colleague had set the filtration on a syringe driver too high, bringing about the premature death of a terminally ill patient? We might like to apply the same repeatable/unrepeatable distinction which was used in the previous example, advising her to speak out only if she believed that her colleague is liable to repeat his mistake.

However, this decision is not without risks. It is not difficult to imagine that the first in anyone's long line of eventually discovered mistakes was perceived at the time to have been a one-off. Likewise, amassing decisive evidence of someone's incompetence is a matter of balancing the effects of a premature claim against the harm that he may inflict over the period that the evidence is amassing.

Summary

The aim of this chapter was to raise questions about what leads us to commend honesty and avoid dishonesty. It is impossible to give hard and fast advice about when dishonesty may be justified, if indeed it ever is. It has also been suggested on at least some occasions when we 'fudge the truth' there is nothing to choose between this and lying, even though our prohibitions against dishonesty are generally phrased in terms of lying, and our commendations of honesty couched in terms of truth-telling. It is important to recognise that a good deal of dishonesty can be promoted through evasion, silence and even truth-telling. At the same time, it is important to recognise that our obligation to be honest does not extend to giving unsolicited advice or opinion, and neither is honesty always promoted by bluntness. Honesty is not simply about being prepared to disclose the truth: some people are not entitled to it, as all bound by a duty of confidentiality know. Allowing patients to accept or take responsibility for their own actions is difficult enough when they are only harming themselves, it is even more difficult when the wellbeing of others is at stake.

In this chapter, the issue of honesty has been addressed almost exclusively as though it is the burden of practitioners. We should not forget, as Farsides (chapter 5) also reminds us, that patients are also moral agents with their own moral burdens, honesty included.

One of the tensions of being a professional is generated by the recognition that one's own actions may have adverse consequences for the profession as a whole. Although I agree with the sentiment that honesty is a stable character trait that permits exceptions and discretion, the repercussions of dishonesty may resonate further afield than we anticipate. This is particularly true in palliative care which has a commendable history of investing considerable effort into treating dying patients openly and honestly.

References and bibliography

Bakhurst D. (1992). On lying and deceiving. *J Med Ethics*, 18(2), 63-6.

Draper H. (1997). Confidentiality. *Journal of the Medical Defence Union,* 13(2), 28-30.

Jackson J. (1991). Telling the truth. *J Med Ethics*, 17(1), 5-9.

Jackson J. (1993). On the morality of deception – does method matter? A reply to David Bakhurst. *J Med Ethics,*19(3), 183-7.

Randell F, Downie RS. (1996). *Palliative Care Ethics: A Good Companion*. Oxford: Oxford University Press.

Todd C, Still A. (1993). General practitioners' strategies and tactics of communication with the terminally ill. *Fam Pract*, 10(3), 268-76.

CHAPTER FOUR

Advocacy

Patricia Webb

Patricia Webb is a Principal Lecturer in Palliative Care at St George's Hospital Medical School and Trinity Hospice, London. Having initially trained as a nurse and become fascinated with cancer, she became interested in multiprofessional education and research, in which she has been involved for several years. Her MPhil research was comparing and contrasting palliative care in the wider Europe with particular emphasis on the interpretation of the ethos underpinning the specialty. She teaches ethics in a variety of educational programmes and is currently a member of a European Commission Europe-wide project on ethical issues in palliative care. She is Editor of the *European Journal of Cancer Care*.

The word 'advocacy' is much used in healthcare but clearly the assumptions and definitions of the users vary. Advocacy is more usually attributed to the practice of law, where the lawyer acts 'on behalf' of the client using expertise that the client does not have. This arrangement is paid for – either directly or through some kind of legal aid.

This exchange of money for professional services significantly alters the balance of power in a professional/client relationship. Whereas the client does not have the required expertise, he does have means of payment for it. In principle therefore, if he does not like what he is buying he can go elsewhere or complain about the service he is getting.

This relationship – of client without expertise paying for a professional to advise – on the whole seems effective. The power acquired through knowledge (in the example quoted) can be accessed and help can be given. There is an acknowledgement that the law is complicated and difficult to interpret without the training to do so.

PROFESSIONAL/LAY RELATIONSHIPS IN HEALTHCARE

In healthcare things are different for a variety of reasons. Of course there is a professional/client (or patient) relationship for the same reasons as the example above but, certainly within a state or nationalised health service where payment is made from general or hypothecated taxes unlinked in time to the professional/lay consultations, there are fundamental differences in the nature of the relationship compared with that of the previous example.

Until fairly recently, probably since the middle 1980s, there continued to be a generally paternalistic approach to healthcare by professional health carers. Some would say that it is still present. The skilled professional takes on a considerable advisory, persuasive or even coercive role with the patient and family. This has generally been the accepted way to proceed and so the actors play out their parts: the professional directs and the client complies. Doctors are asked to advise based on their clinical expertise and examination, aided by investigations and tests. They propose a course of action based on their clinical experience, original knowledge-base and hopefully current evidence-base. The patient and relatives have traditionally not challenged this advice too much but have passively accepted that this is the best current advice available, particularly if the centre from which the clinician works is well regarded.

Nevertheless, there has been some change in this way of working in parts of Europe, as patients have become more informed about health issues and more assertive in their interaction with health professionals. This increase in acquired information has resulted from greater accessibility for the general public to the traditional media sources, now being rapidly complemented by more published work, computer programmes, CD-Rom and websites. These sources are now widely used by a wide range of socio-economic groups in Europe. Those not familiar with more recent technology rely on public libraries or health helplines through the variety of voluntary and other non-governmental organizations that provide these services.

In countries where payment is made at source for any and all healthcare – the United States of America for example – the relationship between doctor (and in some instances other health professionals) and patient is fundamentally different from that within a nationalised health service. There, patients will 'shop around' for healthcare as for any other commodity. For some this will mean shopping within a restricted budget if their health insurance is at basic level. Others will be more privileged and not have such budgetary restrictions. Observation of patients confidently using this system is remarkable in contrast to most of Europe where national health systems are more usual if not inevitable.

For example, in the United States many of those who have not been formally educated and who may have no regular employment are well able to negotiate the best package of healthcare given their circumstances and they do so with great confidence. They have control over the way they use their insurance and so exert a degree of power in their interaction with health professionals.

In the United States the relationship between the value and cost of healthcare and the direct payment for it at the time of delivery, contrasts with the culture in most of Europe of knowing that healthcare will be provided because taxes have been paid as a matter of routine. The direct costs of each package of healthcare are never known in these circumstances.

So, there is an important relationship between client and professional in healthcare. It appears to be influenced by power and status on one part of the relationship compared with relative powerlessness on the other. However, the example quoted of observation of patients in the United States suggests that the relationship need not necessarily be influenced by intellectual ability, poverty or deprivation (although that would vary perhaps, dependent on health culture and policies), providing that payment is part of the direct transaction. The payment for care given reduces the imbalance of power.

Before moving on to look at the role of and possible need for advocacy within healthcare (and in palliative care in particular), it may be helpful to look at some definitions.

Definition of terms

POWER

The term 'power' has been used already several times. It may be defined as:

the ability to do or act; to have the authority to influence another person or organization; to have the ability to control and have superiority or, to have an advantage over others.

The classic discussions and debates on power can be found in the writings of the sociologist Weber. Interested readers should pursue his and others' writings on this phenomenon. (Weber, 1968)

Power may be inappropriately assigned. The power may be conferred by others on an individual without them being able to handle it or without credibility for having it. In that case, inappropriate persuasive or coercive behaviour may result. Constructive use of power comes from real ability and the credibility for achieving it.

In the context of healthcare, power may be acquired because of an exclusive or peculiar knowledge-base (on aspects of healthcare) resulting in prestige and authority of the holder of that knowledge. Webb has alluded to this in the context of professional/patient interactions in oncology (Webb, 1988). She described the imbalance of power between the two parties as a 'social distance' resulting from relative lack of knowledge on one side, with inevitable powerlessness, and expert knowledge on the other side and the power that results from this. Further, the person with expert knowledge uses techniques (whether overtly or covertly) to restrict any possible understanding by the patient or client through use of professional language, jargon and abbreviations. Equal communication between the two is therefore impossible.

It is the observation of this kind of interaction that appears to have persuaded nurses and others that the role of advocacy is needed. Within palliative care there is the assumption that the majority of patients and families feel very vulnerable and unable to articulate their needs. There is little evidence in practice to confirm such assumptions.

It is difficult to consider power and authority without looking at the trait, charisma, particularly within the palliative care context. It has played a considerable role in the establishment and success of the palliative care movement.

Bryman addresses the notion of charisma and leadership, establishing that charismatic leaders can be a great force for good (Bryman, 1992). Those who use their ability to persuade for what the majority perceive as 'good' are exemplified by some of the characters in palliative care. Probably the most well known of these is one of the founder members of the movement, Dame Cicely Saunders. She helped to establish and has continued to feed the development of the modern hospice movement and has assisted in moulding the shape of it within the healthcare context (du Boulay, 1984). There are several others well known in other parts of Europe and further afield who have subsequently demonstrated similar levels of dedication and commitment to palliative care. Charismatic leaders have been a distinguishing feature of successful palliative care developments.

The combination of gentleness and wisdom, supported by experience and a zeal to achieve the goal, has been to the movement's great advantage. Other exemplars of this kind of commitment and gift have been seen repeatedly in the cancer context as well. The most notable example in the UK the establishment of one of the several cancer information organizations, BACUP (now known as 'Cancer Bacup'). Its founder was a female cancer patient who was also a medical scientist and who was driven to remedy what she saw as a huge deficit in the provision of adequate information and support for those with cancer. She achieved an incredible amount before she died from her cancer. This was only possible because of the charisma that enabled her to make others believe in and support her cause and her own zeal to achieve her goals.

The word 'charisma' stems from the Greek for 'grace'. Many would say that charisma may also be a trait of divine inspiration. The goal is always for good. Persuasion, which may be seen as a positive trait as indicated above, may also be a negative trait of the potential or actual dictator. Persuasion without grace is usually negative and it too exists in all facets of life, including healthcare. The goal is then never achieving good but involves a variety of motives which include the glorification of the person rather than the cause.

ADVOCACY

From the moral philosophers' stance advocacy has been defined in the healthcare context as the professional having a role in acting or speaking on behalf of an individual patient or group because of their knowledge, power and influence (in healthcare systems). The goal is to satisfy the interests of the patient, not the professional. General practitioners and nurses in particular seem to see advocacy as one of their clinical tasks. There is a distinct notion of paternalism or maternalism that remains here – for good or bad.

Advocacy simply describes the role of one with expertise who is invited in to negotiate on behalf of another. The important word here is 'invited'. Advocacy on behalf of patients needs to be by their invitation or agreement and should not be an imposition.

There is frequently some confusion between the meaning of 'advocacy' and 'protection' (Webb, 1989). Some have suggested that women are more likely to feel the need to protect patients than men and, in some way, be a surrogate mother or carer to them and to become their advocate. This has certainly been the argument used in the older nursing literature to explain the dependency encouraged by nurses once patients are admitted to hospital. Changing values in western societies however, are reflected in current concerns for the patient's right to know and their right to choice and self-determination in healthcare (Thompson, Melia and Boyd, 1994). Some of the nursing practices have encouraged dependence of patients when it would be more realistic to encourage independent behaviour and to work with patients as partners in care. For patients with serious, life-threatening illness there will be episodes of complete dependence on carers just because patients are too unwell to manage on their own. However, it does seem unrealistic in the long term for a patient not to face the fact of a serious illness: no one can alter the fact of the illness but professional and lay carers can be alongside the patient in the difficult times in their journey. Support is facilitative; encouraging dependency is debilitating.

If one accepts the argument of women wanting to protect, then there is more chance that palliative care patients may be discouraged from independence. Despite the increasing numbers of male nurses, females still predominate. In addition there is a high proportion of female doctors attracted to working in palliative care.

Allen considered this predominance of females in her paper of 1988. She was investigating the career patterns of female doctors and confirmed that they are attracted to and achieve highly in four main specialties: general practice, anaesthetics, psychiatry and radiology. Most doctors attracted to palliative medicine move either from oncology or general practice; oncology, because the majority of patients in palliative care services are still those with advanced cancer. Whilst this is gradually changing so that palliative care includes anyone with a progressive, life-limiting illness, advanced cancer is still the main diagnostic group. The move of doctors between general practice and palliative care is partly accounted for by the increasing needs of palliative care patients at home and partly because the ethos of care for general practice and palliative medicine are considered to be similar. The reasons why women in particular are interested in these areas of work may be because of the flexibility of the work and the early financial security of posts. Ward comments that female doctors are more likely to remain in their chosen specialty than their male counterparts – again for the security and flexibility provided (Ward, 1982). These trends have continued and increased.

There seems to be an assumption that those who are seriously ill will not want to make their own decisions. The evidence from practice is contrary to this. The mind of those facing a life threat is very focused on the life that is left and how to use it. However, as in all aspects of life, there will be those who are strong spirited and independent and those who, through no fault of their own, have learned to be passive and dependent. Both kinds of people and all the variations in between will of course be part of the palliative care setting.

Advocacy in palliative care

Is it necessary even to consider the use of advocacy in palliative care? If so, in what circumstances?

During the patient's passage through the healthcare system, from the first primary healthcare consultation to palliative care, one can observe the kinds of interactions described earlier where there is an imbalance of power and communication is not effective as a result of this.

The simplest way to determine how best to help palliative care patients is to first reduce the degree of vulnerability that they feel in the presence of professionals. The vulnerability is felt more strongly if patients are not on their home ground. This is avoided if patients are seen in their own homes.

If not, all of the well validated communication skills should be used to encourage dialogue: keep with the patient's agenda and not enforce the professional's, take care to provide the most conducive environment to talk and avoid the use of jargon and a patronising attitude.

Then a contractual alliance should be encouraged and fostered. (See also Chapter 5, Farsides.) Establishing the patient's understanding and asking what information they need, does not require highly sophisticated techniques – just concern for another human being and an empathy with how they may be feeling. Given that the main outcome for palliative care is the best possible quality of life remaining, one is looking to provide that which will contribute most to their wellbeing or overall good. Randall and Downie speak of this as the patient's 'total good' (Randall and Downie, 1996).

Only the patient knows what is the best for them, except in cases of emotional and mental confusion and/or dysfunction when they may be unsure what they want and need. Relatives and friends may assume that they know, but what may be a reasonable assumption in health may not be so in ill health.

Relying on a friend or relative to determine what a patient may want or need is a particularly difficult dilemma.

In the palliative care context the professional carer is there to assess and provide both medical and other care. They determine what this care is as well as assessing its 'success'. However, the ideas and ideals of professional and informal carers may differ significantly and any standard care packages may need to be challenged and tailored to individual situations and needs. Making incorrect assumptions may be the greatest block to innovative, individualised care in this field.

In practice, patients have little power to influence the nature of care provision unless a determined effort is made to reduce their actual and perceived vulnerability. To guard against the danger of these comments suggesting almost a conspiracy on the part of the professionals to retain control, it has to be said firmly that the philosophy within palliative care is all about doing the patient good and not controlling or dominating him. However, whilst the motivation and intention may be good, achieving the goal is a different story and regular attention needs to be paid to this.

The professional may have more than one goal: to achieve good for the particular patient, to achieve the goals for all patients, to achieve their own ambitions to provide good palliative care. However, for the patient their only goal is for themselves with perhaps some concern for how this will affect their relatives. Their focus is quite different.

Palliative care patients can feel very vulnerable, frightened and anxious and may well need help to articulate these feelings. They may also need to be given permission to express these feelings without considering that it is weak or stupid to do so. Enabling patients to talk freely about their fears and concerns and accepting that some may not want to talk about their intensely private feelings, is one of the skills of palliative care practitioners. Balancing the power in any interaction will facilitate this. In the circumstances, apart from asking patients if they need the professional to speak on their behalf to a third party, no assumptions need or should be made expecting that to be the case. Whilst patients do have a crisis to deal with in their lives, most of them have come through many crises already in relation to their illness. Many build up a great resilience to this state and, whilst no one can deny the distress, the majority of human beings can deal with the stress that life-threatening illness causes, providing that they have intelligent and caring people supporting them.

There is another side to the story, but it affects the minority only. There will be those who, for a variety of reasons, may need someone to speak on their behalf or to represent their views and ideas to a third party. These will include those patients/clients with a learning disability, the confused, those with a functional communication problem and in some circumstances, the mentally ill and, of course, children. In these instances it seems perfectly reasonable for the professional to ask if the patient would like them or a relative to speak for them in some way and to act as an arbiter between them and a third party. Experience suggests that most but not all are able to answer the question.

For the remaining few, healthcare professionals may have to work with nearest relatives or friends. This is a difficult task and an onerous one for both professionals and relatives. Assumptions of what a patient may want and need are frequently incorrect and may not be the patient's wishes at all. In these circumstances it is always helpful to plan as far ahead as possible with relatives or guardians and to anticipate and rehearse issues likely to arise in the future which may require advocacy skills.

In summary, taking the main outcome of palliative care as achievement of the best possible quality of life left, patients need the real opportunity to speak for themselves. This is facilitated first by the professional's skill in reducing the communication and social gap in any interactions. Second, by asking competent patients if they need help, and having the grace to accept it when they decline, trusting them to know what is best for them. Third, with those who are less able to speak for themselves, again to ask if they need help but if no answer is forthcoming, to check with their closest relatives to try to agree with them the best course of action. This may or may not include the professional acting as an advocate. Finally, assuming that patients always need or want the professional to act as an advocate is unhelpful at least and arrogant at worst and in my experience is infrequently required.

Case 1

A 68-year-old man, Mr B, suffering with chronic obstructive pulmonary disease was referred to specialist palliative care services with severe dyspnoea, cardiac failure and exhaustion. As a widower, his sister was his main carer, but she also had some health problems.

Mr B had lived with deteriorating health for nearly 20 years. He knew his body and he knew that it was finally failing him. There were many signs to convince him of this. Because of his considerable distress resulting from air hunger and poor blood oxygenation, the nurses who received him into the palliative care centre were concerned to do all they could to relieve his symptoms.

Some relief from the dyspnoea and its effects was much appreciated by Mr B. However, he had begun to be irritated by what he described as 'fussing over me' and the suggestions made by nurses that he should change his own practices for survival and comfort that had worked for him for many years and had been appropriately adapted as the disease progressed. Nurses interpreted his irritation as one of the effects of low oxygen levels and acted without his permission by asking a relaxation therapist and the psychologist to see him.

DISCUSSION

These two referrals inflamed the situation and distressed Mr B considerably. Because of his anger it was some days before he was able to articulate his feelings and reveal the mistrust that had resulted from these actions. Far from enhancing his quality of life, these incidents had only served to increase his anxiety, irritation and loss of self-esteem. He thought that he was managing life quite well and only needed help with the medical problems. The nurses' actions undermined his autonomy and reduced his self-esteem and independence. Assumptions were made with no attempt to include him in the discussions about his medical condition and his feelings.

Case 2

Miss P, a 46-year-old woman with rapidly developing multiple sclerosis (MS) was referred for palliative care services with particular reference to neuropathic pain and increasing weakness. A keep-fit fanatic all her life, she had been diagnosed two years previously and was now unable to walk, had no bladder control and reduced bowel control and had considerable anxiety about her body image.

Miss P had not married. She had had a successful career as a high ranking officer in the civil service. Her long-term boyfriend at the time of the diagnosis was unable to deal with the rapid changes in her appearance and her increasing weakness. He left her after a few months.

Since the considerable deterioration in her health, she had employed a nurse and a housekeeper to help her at times during the week but she was still able to do much for herself.

Discussion

There were many opportunities seen by staff to help this woman, not least the challenge to deal with the neuropathic pain in her pelvic floor, radiating to her back and thighs.

A young male doctor took her history when she attended the day centre of a hospice for assessment of her symptoms. Through speaking with this woman for nearly two hours he was able to determine her fiercely independent spirit and yet her total distress at what was happening to her which was outside her control. He had only experienced patients with MS as a very junior house officer and had learned very quickly that there was 'nothing to be done for these poor people'. He had never made an assessment himself of what might be possible or realised that in healthcare there was no such category as 'these poor people', only individuals each with their own story.

Together they made a plan for the following two weeks as follows:

- The traditional remedies for neuropathic pain would be tried for a few days. If these failed to address the problem after a week, referral to an anaesthetist with nerve block and similar skills would be pursued.

- There would be discussion with the physiotherapist to consider hydrotherapy treatment either at the local hospital or possibly at one of the local MS respite centres. Regular attendance might relieve the muscle spasm and fatigue and replace some of the pleasure from exercise that had been lost over the past two years and was yearned for now. If the travel efforts outweighed the benefits then this might not be helpful but it was considered well worth pursuing.

- To combine the expertise of physiotherapy and complementary therapies to address the body image changes experienced by this lady.

- To make a referral to the social worker to discuss possible adaptations to her house so that she could recommence some work in a freelance capacity with possible additional computer skills training and the like.

The initial appearance of this woman into the day centre had been of a young woman with deteriorating health causing many changes in the way she lived and felt. The compassionate and enterprising work of the doctor enabled that rather negative situation to be considerably changed in the space of a couple of hours. This was only possible because of his own open mind and rejection of past prejudices for this particular illness. It was also possible because two adults sat down together and made an alliance to make the best out of this difficult situation and to achieve the main aim of palliative care – the best quality of the life left. Miss P did not need an advocate but someone to give her the access she needed to services that might help her. In effect what was needed was the reduction of the 'social distance' described earlier.

References

Allen I. (1988). Doctors and their careers. In: *Policy Studies Research Report* 675 pp. 246-383. Policy Studies Institute, London.

du Boulay S. (1984). *Cicely Saunders: The Founder of the Modern Hospice Movement.* London: Hodder and Stoughton.

Bryman A. (1992). *Charisma and Leadership in Organisations.* London: Sage Publications.

Randall F, Downie RS. (1996). *Palliative Care Ethics: A good companion.* Oxford: Oxford University Press.

Thompson IE, Melia KM, Boyd KM. (1994). *Nursing Ethics.* 3rd Edition. Edinburgh: Churchill Livingstone.

Ward L. (1982). *People First.* The King's Fund Centre, London.

Webb PA. (1988). Teaching patients and relatives. In: Webb PA. (Ed). *Oncology for Nurses and Healthcare Professionals.* 2nd Edition Vol 2 Care and Support. Beaconsfield: Harper and Row.

Webb PA. (1989). The nurse's viewpoint on ethics. In: Stoll BA. (Ed). *Ethical Dilemmas in Cancer Care.* London: Macmillan.

Weber M. (1968). In: Roth G, Wittich C. (Eds.) *Economy and Society.* New York: Bedminster.

CHAPTER FIVE

How informed can consent be?

Calliope Farsides

Dr Calliope (Bobbie) Farsides is Senior Lecturer in Medical Ethics at the Centre of Medical Law and Ethics, King's College, London. Prior to joining King's in 1996 she was Director of the Centre of Contemporary Ethical Studies at Keele University, and co-founder of their course in the Ethics of Cancer and Palliative Care. She is currently directing a European Commission funded project on *European Palliative Care: Ethics and Communication*. She has published many articles on issues relating to the ethics of palliative care, and is on the editorial board of the *European Journal of Cancer Care*. She is a member of the Ethics group of the National Council for Hospice and Specialist Palliative Care Services.

Consent is a positive buzzword within healthcare vocabulary. There is usually assumed to be a strong moral case for acquiring the consent of the patient, even in those areas where the legal imperative is not decisive. It is important however, to ask why consent is valued in this way, and to enquire as to the role it is meant to play in protecting and pursuing the good of the patient. It is also important to make clear what is required for consent truly to have been given, and to assess in the light of this whether there may be cases in which it is justifiable to work with something other than a clear expression of the patient's consent.

It is a regrettable fact that, from the patient's perspective, consent is often understood primarily as a legal mechanism designed to protect the interests of doctors. It is possible that this understanding will become increasingly prevalent given the growing rates of litigation within the health service. Of course consent does serve a legal function, and part of that function is to protect carers against claims that they have acted without permission, thereby becoming liable for an action in battery, or that they have failed to disclose crucial information, thereby laying themselves open to a claim of negligence. There have been a number of landmark cases involving consent, and many believe that the decisions therein have supported the doctor's position over that of the patient. When a respected legal commentator such as Professor Margaret Brazier concludes that in terms of legal attitudes to consent 'the English courts seem to say that patients must accept and acquiesce in a degree of medical paternalism many enlightened doctors now reject', (Brazier, 1992) it becomes apparent that on this issue at least the law and morality might require different standards of practice.

For this reason it would be more useful for present purposes to consider consent not primarily as a legal concept but as a moral one. Raanon Gillon has provided a very useful definition which manages to capture the essential moral features of a valid consent. According to Gillon consent is:

... a voluntary uncoerced decision made by a sufficiently competent or autonomous person, on the basis of adequate information and deliberation, to accept rather than reject some proposed course of action which will affect him or her. (Gillon, 1986)

By defining consent in this way Gillon draws attention not only to the type of individual who can reasonably be expected to participate in a consenting process (i.e. a sufficiently competent person) but he also specifies the type of decision they must reach (i.e. a voluntary and deliberate choice) and the basis upon which this should be reached (i.e. in the light of adequate information, after careful deliberation, and in the absence of any form of coercion). This definition therefore places demands on carers, institutions and patients. The carer must impart sufficient information and refrain from any words or deeds which might coerce the patient or erode their voluntariness. The institution must allow sufficient time and resources to facilitate the provision of information, and provide the opportunity for reflection and deliberation. The patient must listen to the information provided, and reach a decision. However, there are many ways in which this ideal might be difficult to achieve.

Coercion

Let us consider first the possibility of coercion. To use an extreme example, it would be one thing for me to ask you to agree to giving me a large sum of money whilst we were sitting together over a friendly dinner, and quite another if I (as a stranger) were to do so with a gun pointed at your head. In the first case you would probably respond to my rather unexpected request by asking me why I needed the money, and would then decide whether to give it to me, based on an evaluation of my reasons and of our friendship. In the second case you would simply respond to my threat, fearing the consequences of not doing so.

This might at first appear miles away from a medical or nursing scenario but in many ways the comparison can hold. In some care settings the request for consent will be made in a way which encourages questions, gives time for reflection, and allows the patient to decline. In others a rushed and unfriendly approach will leave the patient feeling they have no choice but to agree. The context in the sense of the physical building and arrangements might also have an effect, just as the open restaurant is quite different to a dark alley. When a person is physically comfortable and at ease they are far less likely to be intimidated or coerced into agreeing to something they are unhappy with. If on the other hand they are embarrassed, uncomfortable, intimidated or distressed by their surroundings their autonomy may well be compromised. However, the most important contextualizing issue is that of the relationship between the carer who requests consent and the patient. If a friend asks me to agree to something I have an understandable context within which to place the request. If a stranger asks me to agree to something I have no such terms of reference. This is an issue which merits further attention.

To place importance on the notion of consent is to characterise the relationship between patient and carer in a particular way. Of course it would not be helpful to employ the friend analogy too forcibly, but it is important to understand that some elements of that type of relationship need to be present, most obviously trust, reciprocity and beneficence. One way to represent these ideas is to present the relationship between carer and patient as contractual, not in the legal sense, but rather in the moral sense which implies the mutual recognition of a set of reciprocal duties and obligations, adopted in the interests of pursuing shared goals. The thinking goes something like this.

By consenting to be my patient you accept that there are certain things that I may expect to do to you, and ask of you, that others would or could not. I make these claims only because we have entered a contract designed to facilitate our

shared goal of pursuing your good and promoting your interests. However,
simply agreeing to be my patient does not settle the consent issue once and for
all. Whilst it might be taken as a tacit permission for certain procedures and
interventions, others will require your express consent, given or withheld after
a specific consideration of the matter at hand.

Sometimes this consent will have a distinctly legal complexion to it, for example
if you require surgery, but on other occasions it will be a matter of personal
negotiation and understanding between you and I, for example when deciding
between various treatment options. Your consent is a sign of your trust in me. My
request for consent is a sign of my respect for you and your autonomy.

There are a number of features of this account which require further
attention. First, the technical distinction that is often made between
express and tacit consent. To consent expressly is to clearly indicate
verbally or perhaps in writing that you agree to a proposed course of
action. This is the clearest sign of consent, although one has to resist
the idea that a verbal or written declaration is always a true sign of
consent. A signature on the end of a form which has been given in the
absence of any explanation, for example, is not consent as morally
understood. Similarly a verbal agreement given by someone too
intimidated to contradict the views of the doctor is not consent in the
way we wish to understand it here.

Because tacit consent is less clear cut in terms of its expression, it is
more open to misinterpretation, or rather we are sometimes too
ready to assume its existence. Often we work with the assumption
that we are entitled to assume that consent has been given when
patients appear to cooperate, or at least do not complain. However,
there is a level of debate over what sort of actions indicate consent in
this way, and how much we can allow to be covered by tacit rather
than express consent.

When I enter a doctor's surgery it may be assumed that I tacitly consent to answer basic questions about my health state which will facilitate a diagnosis, but it should not also be assumed that I tacitly consent to remove all my clothes without an explanation of why this is necessary, nor would it be taken as consent for an invasive procedure such as a biopsy. However, this is not to suggest that express consent is only required for invasive or unusual practices; it may be the case that current practices which appear innocuous and maybe even trivial would benefit from being re-evaluated in the light of a discussion of consent.

Consider the following analogy which hopefully highlights the dangers of assuming too much. If you went to the bank to cash a cheque and handed over your cheque card which had printed upon it your full name – Mr James Bowlby – you would be somewhat surprised if the teller handed it back to you saying 'There you go Jimmy, be a good boy and take it over to the cashier at desk number four'. Convention dictates that when names are used in such a setting formal titles are appropriate.

However, if you find yourself in a hospital bed, hospital staff from the consultant through to the ward orderly may feel entitled to call you by whatever diminutive or pet name they choose. Some patients will be unconcerned or maybe even comforted by this level of informality. Others will find it demeaning and invasive, and interpret it as a lack of respect. The point is that the convention is at odds with ordinary practice and it has the potential to upset or insult the patient, yet rarely if ever will the question of how you wish to be addressed be raised.

It would appear that in this case it is wrong to assume tacit consent, and that the issue of how one is addressed needs to be negotiated and the patient's preference respected. Perhaps this seems a trivial point but consider it from the opposite perspective. Imagine the surprise of the eminent consultant Professor Patricia Callow who suddenly gets beckoned across the ward by the new patient in bed number four shouting 'Hey Trish, can you toddle over here love?'. It is highly likely that this encounter will colour the relationship that develops from there on between carer and patient, but without knowing something of the character and preferences of the Professor we cannot predict whether those effects will be good or bad. In practice the prevailing conventions will make such an encounter unlikely; the patient on the other hand is subject to conventions which can lean towards what they might consider patronizing and irritating familiarity.

The underlying rule is this: tacit consent should be taken to mean the same as express consent, with only the mode of expression being different. Some conventions will be so widely accepted and acceptable that tacit consent to their adoption can be assumed, and the onus would be on the patient to ask that something different should happen. However, in the example cited here we should remain wary of tacit consent.

If we were to transport the widely acceptable convention of addressing people formally on first meeting into the hospital ward, some people would feel happy to say 'Please call me Jim' if that is what they preferred, others would not but would nonetheless feel uncomfortable with the formality, or perhaps take it to be representative of a gap between patient and carer that does not in reality exist.

Far better surely to negotiate with the patient at the outset: 'Mr Bowlby, welcome to Ward Ten, I'm Nurse Jones but please call me Rachel if you prefer. Tell me, how would you like to be addressed while you are here?'. This will hopefully mark the beginning of the type of relationship required for the proper working of the contractual model of care.

Sufficient information

Another feature of Gillon's definition that obviously requires attention is the issue of 'sufficient information'. This is commonly understood to imply a responsibility on the part of the carer to impart information to the patient.

However, before considering this more familiar aspect of the issue, it is worth looking at it in a slightly different way. A morally defensible consenting process also requires the carer to collect or receive sufficient information from the patient.

The contractual model which is presented here is predicated upon the assumption of shared goals. This is not contentious at a very general level. We can make assumptions that the patient wants to be helped by the carer and that the carer wishes to help the patient. But of course we also need to verify that the goals are not only shared in this general way, but also that they are understood in the same way when it comes to specifics. For example, what type of help does the patient require, what type of help is the carer capable of offering, what type of help is he prepared to offer?

This is a particularly important issue within the context of palliative care, where the carer will possibly play a major role in what is left of the patient's life and indeed their death. A patient may have particular ideas about how they wish to live the rest of their life, how they want to die and so on, and these beliefs and attitudes will be an expression of their autonomy.

By understanding consent as an ongoing procedure rather than a number of single events, one facilitates the discovery of these goals and attitudes. To know that a patient still consents to the care they are receiving requires an ongoing dialogue about and around that care and the goals it is designed to achieve. It also requires that the carer provide the patient with information, assess their satisfaction, and listen to what they are being told. Prior to engaging in this dialogue the carer may have a very clear idea of their professional role, what they are required to do for their patient and what they are unprepared to do. But the carer's attitudes might also have to be modified in the light of a new understanding of the goals that this particular patient has set, and the way in which this particular person evaluates the quality and value of their life.

During the course of this dialogue there may be moments when matters become complicated if, for example, the patient requests something the carer feels unable to provide, or the patient refuses something the carer feels obliged to offer and inclined to promote. However, the best chance of resolving these issues surely lies with establishing a full understanding between patient and carer of the goods which each is seeking to pursue. Ideally this shared knowledge would facilitate a level of tolerance and understanding which would on occasions allow one party to consent to or refuse something which is nonetheless at odds with their basic ideas.

So, for example, in exploring a patient's reasons for refusing treatment a physician might come to understand and thereby accept that this choice is appropriate for the patient given their assessment of their quality of life, their sense of personal identity, and their preferences regarding the manner and time of their death. The carer could therefore consent to the patient's request not to be treated by various means even if they themselves remained convinced that the patient's life could be maintained at a decent quality. Similarly, the patient could come to understand why the carer wanted to continue in a particular way.

Other cases might be more difficult. Consider the following four cases and make your own assessments.

CASE 1

Dillon is a traveller who hit the road three years ago, shortly after his diagnosis of testicular cancer. His philosophy on life is highly individualistic and his past refusal of treatment means that an essentially treatable cancer has been allowed to spread. He is now in severe pain and has finally approached a local GP who has referred him to you at the local pain control clinic based within the hospice.

Dillon has requested pain control but refuses to accept the particular drugs you are recommending because he claims they are made by a 'particularly immoral' pharmaceutical company. You believe that the company is no worse than any other, in fact in many respects they have a good record. However, you trust that Dillon will not have any knowledge of a smaller company that produces a near equivalent, and although you know them to have been involved in rather shady dealings in the developing world you prescribe their drug and keep quiet. Dillon agrees to take the drugs.

DISCUSSION

In this example it is probably very difficult for the doctor to understand the patient and share their value systems. However, the doctor appears to find a way to make Dillon feel all right about his actions, even if they are essentially no better than the choice he rejected. His may be the best action in one respect, but we need to ask whether Dillon has really consented or whether his values have been respected. It might be that no drug has yet been produced by means that Dillon considers ethical, and if we were truly to respect his position we would need to allow him to refuse all mainstream therapies.

This would be a very difficult option for many carers to accept, but it would show respect for the autonomy of a patient who would appear to be competent to make decisions about his life and welfare, and the values he wishes to live by.

However, in the past and still to an extent today there has been a readiness on the part of healthcare practitioners to substitute their own perceptions of the good for those of the patient, or to pursue their conception of the goals of medicine unquestioningly assuming them to be universally endorsed. This is essentially paternalism, and one of the functions of consent is to guard against the excesses of paternalism.

In imparting the information necessary to consent, one allows the patient to either share or contradict your view, and if they wish to do so they can make it their own. In discovering important information about the patient one is forced to acknowledge that their world view might be radically different to your own and that this will have consequences for the choices they make.

However, there may be justified forms of paternalism appropriate to the care of particular patients, and a feature of some justifiable forms of paternalism may well be the willingness to act in the patient's best interest irrespective of their consent. This is an issue in the treatment of those judged incompetent to consent. But it might also be an issue where the costs to the patient of being asked to consent are thought to be too great.

CASE 2

Jean is a 42-year-old woman with breast cancer. She is aware of her diagnosis and prognosis, but she has said from the outset that she cannot take responsibility for her treatment in any way. She does not wish to be made to choose between options, rather she wants you to decide on her behalf. She is happy to hear from you why you have made the choices you make, and to that extent she will be fully informed of the situation. In this case, consent has been given for the carer to take complete control of the management of the patient. Jean remains perfectly happy with the arrangement, and devotes her time to sorting out those things she thinks matter most in the time she has left.

DISCUSSION

Such an arrangement places a heavy responsibility on the carers, but it may be one that they should be prepared to accept on behalf of some patients. However, for it to work properly the carers not only need to know all the necessary information about the care they can offer, they also need to know Jean, as that will be the only way to ensure that the choices they make on her behalf are appropriate and, looking at it from the opposite angle, that is what they have consented to do. Some would object to this arrangement as it pays too little attention to patient autonomy, but this need not be the only interpretation.

Consent often indicates trust and allows the patient to hand over control and responsibility without losing autonomy. Autonomy is usually defined and understood in terms of the idea of self rule and is taken to be a particularly valuable feature of humanity which should be promoted and respected. It is thought to be intrinsically good to be master of one's own life, and further extrinsic goods are taken to follow on from this. However, it is important not to confuse autonomy with a crude notion of substantive independence. There are times in one's life when one does not wish to be entirely in control of one's welfare, and in fact no great benefit would follow from being so. Others are the experts on the issue in question, and to hand over some control to them would be of benefit both in terms of securing the best outcome, but also in terms of relieving oneself of responsibilities one might not feel equipped to fulfil.

The crucial term here is 'hand over', and one can add to this the idea of consenting to do so, and monitoring and reassessing one's decision over time. If I consent to allow someone to take control of some important aspect of my life then my autonomy is not eroded, even though my level of independence and control has been. If I employ an expert accountant to take care of my financial affairs I consider this to be quite different to an overbearing partner insisting on doing so. I employ the accountant because of their expertise and understand them to be relieving me of an onerous burden. My partner on the other hand in denying me control without my agreement attacks my autonomy. If the accountant were to decide to take radical action which went beyond the normal duties I understood her to be carrying out, then I might believe that she also is taking too much control and would feel that my autonomy was threatened.

Consent is an ongoing process with only a limited range of activities taken to be tacitly consented to once the original relationship is set up. Not everyone is like Jean, nor should they be treated in the manner she requests. Care should generally be seen as shared rather than delegated, negotiated rather than prescribed.

Many of the features of Gillon's definition underline the importance of time in the consenting process, and lack of time needs to be acknowledged as a potential problem. Time is needed for the patient's competence to be assessed. Time is needed for information to be given, understood and deliberated on. Time is also needed to form the relationship between carer and patient which will protect against the dangers of coercion and unjustified paternalism. And, over time, circumstances relevant to consent can change.

Think about the relationship between a GP and a patient. If you see the same GP from childhood, at a certain point the terms of the relationship need to be re-negotiated. When you are very young your parents act as proxies and give their consent to treatment as required. As you get older they do not need to fulfil this role, and it should not be assumed that you consent to your parents being involved with or even informed of your medical treatment. As you reach old age, or in specific situations beforehand, the need for a proxy might arise again, or at least there might be occasions on which it is wise to keep another person informed of your situation. With this in mind carers will need to constantly check back to establish who are the significant others in the picture and the extent to which, if at all, they may be consulted or informed.

Likewise, in a relationship that exists over time the doctor's understanding of the attitudes and beliefs of the patient need to be reconfirmed over time, and sometimes issues need to be raised and discussed in anticipation of later events or conditions the patient might experience. A GP should not, for example, assume that a child will share the moral beliefs of its parents, nor that a person who was vehemently opposed to something in early life remains similarly committed at a later stage.

But of course few of us enjoy the luxury of continuous care as characterised by the old style family doctor. On the cancer journey our care might pass through many hands and we might confront many different types of institution. Yet at each point along the way it is important for our carers to know who we are, where we have come from and where we wish to go.

An important aspect of early outpatient care might be to discuss with patients issues that are important to their later care management and treatment choices, but also to share with them their understanding of the situation they find themselves in and the continuities and discontinuities with their earlier life.

The key to successful consent throughout the therapeutic relationship lies with the successful establishment and nurturing of the relationship between carer and patient, and the sharing of information, ideas, plans and goals over time. The time available will of course vary, dependent upon when and how a person is diagnosed and what type of care they have access to. Continuity of care over time offers the fullest opportunities for information sharing, understanding and consent but it should be possible for a patient's care to pass successfully through the hands of different people, as long as those carers work together to ensure that the patient experiences the same essential relationship with each.

CASE 3

Rachel has been attending the local hospice as an outpatient for two years since she was first diagnosed with non-Hodgkin's lymphoma. She has seen Ian, the Nurse Manager of the unit, on each of her regular visits. They have discussed many things together, not always matters related to her illness, and Ian has kept a full set of notes documenting what he considers to be significant information emerging from their conversations. At the beginning of each visit Ian shares these notes with Rachel, and she confirms whether they were an accurate account of what was said or understood. Unfortunately Rachel is quite ill now and is confined to her home where Susie, the community nurse, visits her regularly. With Rachel's agreement Susie has read Ian's notes and has discussed them with Rachel on her second visit.

DISCUSSION

Ian's notes give Susie an initial introduction to her patient, and allow Rachel to build a relationship with Susie without having to rebuild the basic foundations. Future consents will be informed by numerous previous discussions between Ian and Rachel, even though Ian is no longer directly involved in her care. The other side of the coin is that Susie has a responsibility to make Rachel feel happy with her, and get to know her in the relatively short time they might have together.

Having moved away from the old misconception that 'there is nothing more we can do' once somebody is found to be terminally ill, there are increasing numbers of therapeutic options available designed to either prolong or improve the quality of that life. However, some of these treatments are in themselves burdensome and it is not always clear that the right choice would be to intervene. However, if such treatments are available and there is at least some chance of improvement, one could say that to fail to disclose the possibility of benefit and offer the patient a choice is unduly paternalistic.

The problem is that in order to facilitate rational choice one has to give the patient all the relevant facts, some of which will be difficult to cope with, others of which can only be presented as possibilities or probabilities. Furthermore, to make choices which affect their future the patient needs to understand what their future holds for them, and that might be knowledge that they have so far chosen to resist acquiring.

The lesson here is that the possibility of choice and the requirement to gain consent requires openness and honesty through the course of the entire relationship between carer and patient. If these have always been features of the relationship between carer and patient, the particular truths that have to be delivered at moments of choice will not come as a shock in the same way as they might when a carer has paternalistically selected what the patient should or should not know.

At the end of life, a person might no longer be able to make decisions or express their consent. This does not mean that there will not be important choices to be made, nor does it mean that consent can or should disappear from the picture.

There are a number of different ways in which consent can still be incorporated in such a patient's care. First, following on from the discussion above, it should be possible for carers and patients to work together and discuss in advance the types of choices a person would want to make in given situations. This is formalised by way of the advance directive or living will.

CASE 4

Robert is a 42-year-old gay man suffering from end stage HIV-related disease. He is blind, barely conscious and mildly demented. However, he can be cared for easily at home and has as yet required no unusual means to keep him alive. His partner David has cared for him devotedly and now feels that it is time for him to die before his dignity is further eroded. Robert's mother agrees and is happy to care alongside David. However, Robert's father and sister feel he should be admitted to hospital so that 'something could be done' were a crisis to occur. Robert has prepared a living will, but actually found that he could live with some of the conditions he previously considered intolerable such as his blindness. Therefore, whilst still competent he chose not to activate it.

DISCUSSION

Such a case hints at the problems associated with remaining true to the moral purpose of consent once a patient is no longer competent. An advance directive is a form of prospective consent expressly given. In such a document the patient will use their legal right to specify what types of treatments and interventions they wish to refuse at what stage in their life. There are a number of difficulties with these documents, and it is rare that they do not require some form of interpretation or endorsement by others. However, combined with an understanding of the patient based on earlier encounters, or through discussion with significant others, it should be possible to ascertain when, if at all, it is appropriate to activate such a document, and thereby let the patient effectively consent whilst non-competent.

Prior to the development of these documents the only options were proxy consent, hypothetical consent (deciding on the basis of what someone would consent to if only they were able), or beneficent management in the interests of the patient. Each of these options raises problems. In the case of Robert we would need to ask who should act as proxy? Is it the person with the firmest legal relationship, or the person closest to and most cognisant of the patient's wishes? Should those who have the clearest legal right to decide necessarily enforce that right against others who would be better qualified to decide on behalf of the patient?

The problem is that all those gathered at the bedside love Robert and want to do what is best for him, and it is difficult to admit that one might not be the best person to judge what precisely that is.

David feels that what is best for Robert at this stage is 'what Robert wants', but Robert is unable to tell us what he wants so we need to work it out. David will do this by referring back to discussions they have had since Robert's diagnosis, by recalling the way he has seen Robert live his life and the plans he knows Robert to have made for his death. The problem is that Robert has already abandoned one of the plans he earlier made, and we have no way of knowing how he feels at the moment.

Robert's father and sister may see the best for Robert as 'more life', and therefore they wish to secure that on his behalf. His mother may see the best for Robert as an end to his pain and suffering irrespective of what he has or has not said in the past.

Deciding what is in the patient's best interests is not the simple task it is presented as when carers suggest that in the absence of consent we should decide in the patient's best interest. For this reason it is in the interest of all those involved to develop the consenting process in ways which allow it to be part of a patient's care even when their competence has vanished, be that through involving the patient at an earlier stage in the appointment and briefing of proxies, or through fine tuning the advance directive mechanism to make it a reliable expression of the patient's wishes.

This chapter has looked at the issue of consent and has indirectly tackled the question of whether it can be fully informed, but it has done so in a rather unexpected way. Of course there are important questions surrounding the issue of how much a patient should be told, when they should be told, how they should be told, and by whom.

There are minimum standards which ought to be met on all these points, and there are moral and empirical arguments to support specific levels of information giving as necessary to appropriate consent. However, all this good work will come to nought if this information is fed into a context which undermines its purpose.

Information, that is the facts when they are available, probabilities or opinions when they are not, is the basic raw material of deliberation and choice. Competence, autonomy and confidence provide the patient with the tools they need to work with that raw material. A strong, open and truthful relationship with their carers affords them invaluable assistance in their task. Most importantly of all, the information the carer gathers about the patient allows her to assist in the task without getting in the way; to take over the task when the patient gets in trouble and asks for help; to carry the burden when the task gets too much for the patient to bear; or to step in when the patient loses the basic skills they need to progress.

It is not always possible to obtain consent, and patients are not always willing to shoulder the responsibilities that are imposed by consent. Eventualities such as these need to be anticipated.

Wherever possible, consent needs to be an ongoing component of care, but so does the free and honest exchange of information. Without the latter the former becomes a sham; without either the patient at best gets lost within a sea of beneficence and at worst is drowned in professional arrogance.

To make a rational choice the patient needs to know the relevant information; to make a free, voluntary and uncoerced choice the patient needs to know and trust her carer. To ensure that consent is given the carer needs to impart information to the patient and gather information about the patient in order to build the relationship that is needed to insure against coercion, intimidation or undue influence. Only when both sides of this contract are fulfilled will consent be fully informed in the way we require it to be.

References

Brazier, M. (1992). *Medicine, Patients and the Law*. London: Penguin Books.

Gillon, R. (1986). *Philosophical Medical Ethics*. London: John Wiley and Sons.

CHAPTER SIX

Euthanasia
slippery slope or mercy killing?

Marney Prouse

Marney Prouse completed a BA in Sociology at the University of Western Ontario and her nursing education was completed at Sault College in Ontario, Canada. She began her palliative care career at the Hospital for Sick Children, Toronto where she was Service Manager for Cystic Fibrosis and Respiratory Diseases and for children with life-threatening conditions. She moved to England in 1990 when she was Director of Nursing and Quality Assurance at Trinity Hospice, London, where she also lectured on law and ethics. She completed a Bachelor of Law degree at the University of Westminster, London and is currently Risk and Litigation Manager at North West Anglia Healthcare Community Trust, Peterborough. She developed the organisational audit for Specialist Palliative Care Services as a joint project with the King's Fund Organisational Audit Unit, working with palliative care units in England, Ireland, Hong Kong and Kenya.

It has long been thought that the process of dying was a fairly straightforward one. Generations before ours were saddened but resigned to death as an inevitable part of life. In the words of Eric Wilkes (1994), one of the stalwarts of the British palliative care movement, death, until recently, was a social act. However, recent years have brought significant changes to the technology that keeps patients alive. The patient of the past, who would have followed a natural progression from illness or injury through to organ failure to death, now has the intervention of technology available in many cases.

David Lamb (1985) writes that while death is an event, dying is a process. We have allowed technology to steer the course of death so that it remains a process rather than a final event and a far cry from the social act it once was. In doing so, we create moral dilemmas for those who would have died in days gone by and who would now choose to die, but find that they would need assistance in so doing.

Few subjects provoke such heated debate as that of euthanasia. The inevitable lines of battle are drawn between those who believe in sanctity of life at all costs and those who believe that individuals who are terminally ill should be free to determine the moment and route of their deaths. The purpose of this chapter is not to determine whether euthanasia is right or wrong, but to arm the reader with some essential ethical arguments that are both critical and challenging. Another aim is to examine some of the most debated arguments and to present some often unacknowledged alternatives to them based on overviews of writings by a number of contributors to the field. This subject has challenged some of the greatest minds through the ages and many books and treatises have been written as a result. This chapter will present a brief overview of some of that thinking and hopefully, will encourage the reader to explore the concepts on a fuller and deeper basis.

The logical starting point for this discussion is to define the concept. This being a complex subject, its definition is by necessity complex and not necessarily universally agreed. Glover (1977) baldly says that euthanasia is used to mean:

killing someone, where, on account of his distressing physical or mental state, this is thought to be in his own best interests. It is to include someone who is about to enter such a state as well as someone who is already there.

Roy and Rapin (1995), writing on behalf of the European Association for Palliative Care, say that the term should be reserved for:

compassion-motivated, deliberate, rapid and painless termination of the life of someone afflicted with an incurable and progressive disease. A suffering and terminally ill person is not allowed to die - his or her life is terminated.

It is often on the basis of such emotive words as killing and termination that discussions on the subject stray into imbalance.

Some further definitions have been advanced in a report published by the House of Lords Sub Committee on Medical Ethics (UK) during which time the sub committee considered evidence on the subject of euthanasia. They sub-divided euthanasia into three further categories.

Voluntary euthanasia identifies that the patient is capable of forming consent and requests his or her own death.

Non-voluntary euthanasia occurs when the patient does not have the capacity to understand what euthanasia means and therefore cannot form a request or withhold consent. This term is most often applied to those patients who are mentally incompetent because they have learning disabilities or those patients who are unconscious and cannot give or withhold consent. Patients such as Karen Ann Quinlan, the young woman in persistent vegetative state (PVS) in the United States whose case made medicolegal history in 1976 (as quoted in Pabst

Battin 1994) or Tony Bland, the young man who was also in PVS for a prolonged period as a result of injuries sustained at the Hillsborough football match disaster in 1993 (UK) are examples of other types of patients for whom permission might be sought by third parties to discontinue treatment that might otherwise prolong their lives. This is certainly the type of patient who receives considerable attention from the press, not least because their cases have two major elements. The first is that third parties seek permission for them to die. The other and, perhaps more critical issue is that these patients cannot give consent because they are deemed to be incompetent. This area will be discussed later in the chapter.

Involuntary euthanasia is the killing of a patient who is capable of understanding and consenting to the act, but does not do so. This may also be known as murder within the ambit of the law.

Assisted suicide describes the act sought by a competent patient who wishes to end his or her life, but requires assistance to perform the act, either because of a physical disability or, as in most cases, because the patient is not armed with sufficient information to ensure that death will be guaranteed. Physician-assisted suicide as described by the American Medical Association (AMA) occurs 'when the physician facilitates a patient's death by providing the necessary means and/or information to enable the patient to perform the life-ending act (e.g., the physician supplies sleeping pills and information about the lethal dose while aware that the patient may commit suicide)' (*Bulletin of Medical Ethics,* 1996).

Passive euthanasia was a term widely used to describe the withholding or withdrawing of life-sustaining treatment by which the patient is allowed to die. The use of the term has fallen foul of the palliative care community who have suggested that the terms 'active' and 'passive' are ambiguous and misleading and so should be avoided.

The House of Lords Select Committee UK (1993) agrees with the European Association of Palliative Medicine and suggests that the terms 'withdrawing or not initiating treatment or... a treatment limiting decision' are more appropriate descriptors. The Dutch have a term 'levesbeeindigend handelen', or life-terminating acts, that encompasses withholding and withdrawing of all treatment and it is used to refer to the direct termination of life as found in the Remmelink Commission Report commissioned by the Dutch Supreme Court in 1991-92 (Pabst Battin, 1994).

THE LEGAL STATUS OF EUTHANASIA

Contrary to popular opinion, until very recently, euthanasia could only be practiced legally in one country in the world. The Northern Territories in Australia was the first state to legalise and sanction the practice of euthanasia in 1996. The first case of euthanasia under that law occurred in September 1996 when a man who was terminally ill was able to commit suicide with the help of the provision of a computer-assisted lethal injection that was prepared by his general practitioner (*BMJ*, 1996). On 24 March 1997, a bill was passed in the Australian parliament that overturned the legality of the decision to allow euthanasia to be practised, now rendering it illegal (*The Guardian*, 25 March 1997).

This was not the first state to legalise euthanasia, but it was the first to sanction its practice. During the short life of this law, four people committed suicide with the help of their doctors. Oregon, a state on the west coast of the United States, legalised the practice of euthanasia in 1995 after a referendum to support its use was held. An immediate challenge to that law occurred and although the law was a valid one, an appeal by opposition groups made the practice illegal immediately. The challenge is still in effect.

One of the most commonly held misconceptions is that The Netherlands holds the title for the longest legalised approach to euthanasia. On the contrary, it is still a crime for a doctor or other healthcare professional to commit euthanasia in Holland, but protection accompanies such an action which is called a defence of necessity, assuming that there has been scrupulous adherence to stringent criteria. Failure to meet the criteria could result in a maximum prison sentence of twelve years.

Changes were made to the law in 1997 which have relaxed some of the criteria, most notably by having cases reviewed by regional committees of doctors, lawyers and ethicists (*BMJ*, 1997). Having said that there is government protection for those doctors who participate in explicit, informed, voluntary euthanasia, it appears that the practice is not widespread, accounting for 1.8% of reported deaths (Pabst Battin, 1994). The government is aware that under-reporting may be an issue and is attempting to document to what extent euthanasia is under-reported. It is examining officially registered cases of assisted deaths and 1,000 randomly sampled deaths as well as court cases in which the wish to die could not be expressed (*Lancet*, 1996).

Despite that, the Dutch Voluntary Euthanasia Society (NVVE) received over 600 telephone complaints after publicising its telephone number in a bid to counterbalance the official government enquiry evaluating the euthanasia guidelines which became law in 1994. One quarter of the callers complained that their doctor would not comply with their wishes and another quarter said that their doctor promised to help them end their lives, but did not. Another quarter found that there were misunderstandings between different doctors caring for the patient. The remainder of the callers said that their doctors hid behind bureaucracy to avoid being involved in the practice of euthanasia (*Lancet*, 1996).

The legal position in the United Kingdom is quite clear: euthanasia is a criminal offence, although the courts have not reacted strongly by failing to convict doctors under the Suicide Act since its introduction in 1961. The relevant bit of law is in section 2(1) of the Act which states it is an offence 'to aid, abet, counsel or procure the suicide of another or an attempt by another to commit suicide'. This does not however, stop charges being laid under the criminal law, the most common being a charge of murder.

An interesting paper reported from Scotland in *The Lancet* suggests that a distinction can be made between euthanasia and the withdrawal of treatment and that the various routes to death that are collectively and, possibly, inaccurately, called euthanasia. In order to resolve that, the paper suggests isolating the various aspects of the term and addressing them within the law. It should be clearly noted here that the law in Scotland is legally separated from that in England and Wales. However, the principle is a sound one. One suggestion is to deal with persistent vegetative state as a separate entity and to propose the introduction of a Medical Futility Bill which has the following wording:

It will not be unlawful to withdraw treatment, including physiological replacement therapy such as artificial ventilation and feeding, when at least two independent registered medical practitioners, one of whom must be a consultant neurologist, are of the opinion that the patient has sustained such damage to the central nervous system that:

- *he cannot exist in the absence of continuous care*

- *he is permanently unable to participate in human relationships and experiences*

- *continued treatment cannot improve this condition and is therefore futile; and*

- *the patient's nearest relatives or carers have been consulted.*

The authors of this proposed bill consider physician-assisted suicide and suggest that as suicide has never been a criminal offence in Scotland, then aiding and abetting a suicide would likely not be a crime in Scotland. A physician who assists a patient to commit suicide in England may possibly be guilty under Section 2(1) of the Suicide Act 1961, although, as stated above, there is no evidence that this would happen. The authors suggest that a section should be added to the Suicide Act that under Section 2, a physician would be excluded from a charge if s/he was a registered medical practitioner who, given the existence of a competent directive, providing assistance to a patient who is suffering from a progressive and irremediable condition and who is prevented, or will be prevented, by physical disability from ending his or her own life without assistance.' (Mason and Mulligan, 1996)

This bears a close resemblance to the conditions under which Dutch doctors have practiced for a number of years and moves one step closer to mediating some of the thornier issues that have faced clinicians and the judiciary. Cases such as Airedale NHS Trust v Anthony Bland (1993) would not necessarily have to be heard in courts and certainly not taken to the highest court in the land.

The information presented above has been fairly straightforward and factual and this presents relatively few obstacles to a debate on euthanasia. The challenges begin when the philosophers and ethicists begin to present their arguments and counter-arguments. Who is right? As noted earlier, it is not possible to make a definitive statement about who is right or who is wrong as each side will present a provocative debate. The task facing the student of ethics is to identify good arguments and those that are flawed. The biggest challenge of all, however, is to recognise that no morally correct solution can be deduced from a single ethical principle. Having said that, some of the principles that may be used to guide us are inherently incompatible

(Spiers, 1997). Some of us wish to debate in the hope that the decision will be less uncomfortable, that the choices will be easier to make. Wishing it was so will not make it easier. However, believing that a balanced viewpoint and well-constructed thinking have been exercised in the discussion of this topic, may assist in feeling satisfied that all that could have been done was done. The following arguments have been heard in some form or another and in some depth or another for many years. This brief space presents the opportunity to identify an introduction to the argument surrounding euthanasia.

THE THREE COMPONENTS TO A DEBATE ON EUTHANASIA

Margaret Pabst Battin (1994), a bioethicist, identifies that it is in serious moral error to oppose euthanasia on the grounds of three fundamental moral principles: mercy, autonomy and justice.

The mercy argument has two essential components. Linked in a peripheral way to the double effect argument discussed later, is the principle of beneficence, which is seen as a duty to prevent or remove harm or a duty to promote good. This duty is best illustrated in palliative care as a duty to act to end pain or suffering already occurring. An alternative consideration to be held is that of non maleficence, a duty not to do harm which thereby forms a core of morality exhorting us not to cause further pain and suffering, not to kill, to disable and so on. These two elements, where a health professional has a duty to balance the principles of beneficence and non maleficence before making decisions about patient care, form the core of the mercy argument.

The health professional might ask such questions as 'is the treatment doing good?', 'is the treatment causing harm to the patient?' or 'is the compliance with the patient's wishes harmful?' to determine the scope of intervention and treatment and to serve as a useful springboard for further discussions with the patient and his or her family. Thus, euthanasia could be considered to be morally right. However, Rachels (1986) develops this further into a more rigorous argument. He suggests that utilitarianism should be examined in the light of actions being right or wrong according to whether they caused happiness or misery. If the actions were judged by this standard, then euthanasia would be morally acceptable. The principle of utility states that any action is morally right if it increases the amount of happiness in the world or if it decreases the amount of misery. The argument then goes on to say that killing, at his or her own request, a terminally ill patient who is suffering intolerably would decrease the amount of suffering in the world, then this action would be morally right. This argument, says Rachels, is much too simplistic to be totally useful as these are not the only morally important things. If that view is expanded to include the ability to maximise one's interests, then Rachels says while the promotion of happiness and avoidance of misery are not the only morally important things, they are important nonetheless, so if an action decreases misery and suffering, then it is one very strong reason in its favour. The theme of incompatible ideals and ideas and of more than one principle being applicable to the argument is beginning to develop. Readers would be well advised to further explore the doctrine of utilitarianism and the principle of utility.

Those opposed to euthanasia say that the mercy argument is misplaced. Gormally (1994) likens euthanasia to putting a sick or injured animal out of its misery: mercy is confused with loving care. He says that 'mercy sustains and supports and you cannot take care of something by destroying it. But you can judge it not worth preserving and sympathy is one of things that can make it feel intolerable to put up with a creature's gross suffering and may even incline one to terminate a reduced and pathetic existence.'

This standpoint is supported by Brock (1994) who brings it within a more realistic framework. He says that the critical premise of the mercy argument is false because there are not great numbers of patients who are suffering, thanks to the advances of palliative care. If patients are suffering, he maintains, it is because there is a 'wrongful failure' to provide adequate pain relief. This is an interesting premise and one on which the palliative care movement depends to actively oppose voluntary euthanasia. This will be discussed later in the chapter.

Another principle to be considered is that of autonomy, defined by Beauchamp and Childress (1979) as 'a concept of self-governance: being one's own person, without constraint either by another's action or by psychological or physical limitations'. The autonomous person determines his or her own course of action in accordance with a plan chosen by himself or herself. Such a person deliberates about and chooses plans, and is capable of acting on the basis of such deliberations. Glover (1990) says that questions of autonomy can only arise in the context of a person who has a preference at the time when a decision is to be taken, which then eliminates the mentally incompetent person from this arena. Faulder (1985) says that at the very heart of autonomy is the concept of respect for persons and, by extension, a respect for the decisions they choose to make and the rights they choose to exercise. Pabst Battin (1994) says that autonomy supports euthanasia: 'one ought to respect a competent person's choices, where one can do so without undue costs to oneself, where doing so will not violate other moral obligations and where these choices do not threaten harm to any persons or parties.'

Pabst Battin suggests that if the threads of the arguments around mercy were picked apart, then every patient with an illness, injury or disability should be able to claim full support for whatever treatment they require, for as long as they require it. Can our society support such a concept? Can our financial and human resources stretch to infinity? Should resources be available to everyone, or only to a select few? Who would choose the few? Knowing that there have been some challenges to this notion, then the principle of justice or fairness must be called into play to mediate and to assist in distributing the limited resources we have.

This is not a theoretical issue. Former British Secretary of State for Health, Virginia Bottomley, said that 'in a modern health service, every clinical decision took place within finite resources' (*Times*, 1995). This might include invoking justice based on the greatest medical need, or who can pay, or whether medical intervention would offer a complete restoration of function, or whose contributions to society have been the greatest. This principle can also assist with decisions to be made for those whose conditions are not self-induced – the non-smoker, the person who does not abuse drugs. Pabst Battin says that it is often argued that if treatment is denied to people with the result that they will die, then is it not better to deny treatment to those who are 'medically unsalvageable' and will die at any rate. This, she says, justifies the practice of euthanasia on the basis of what is known as the salvageability principle – salvaging those who will not die so soon and letting the others die – the terminally ill patient, the defective neonate. Euthanasia is in accord with this principle by the demands of justice in a situation of scarcity of resources. She does warn that denying treatment on the grounds of justice does not strictly qualify as euthanasia, as the denial of treatment is not done to promote a 'good death'. Again, this is a 'taster' for the reader who wishes to explore further the principles of distributive justice and to formulate personal arguments about its use. Questions to ask might be 'does justice provide a smokescreen for treatment-limiting decisions or passive euthanasia', or 'does rationing present risks to our healthcare system?'; 'which criteria might be used to justify euthanasia?'. There are many, many more questions to be asked, but not necessarily answered. The point is to identify many points of view so that balanced thinking and argument is the outcome.

An objection to the argument of justice is the 'slippery slope' argument, so named because it is argued that if we travel down the road of sanctioning euthanasia, then it is one further slide down the slippery slope to uncontrolled and unregulated action. There is widespread belief amongst philosophers and ethicists that the slippery slope argument is illogical and does not bear close scrutiny. The aim of this section is to equip the reader with an overview of critical thinking about the slippery slope argument. Again, this is not an attempt to sway thinking, but to allow the reader a more balanced view on this rather persuasive argument.

Pabst Battin (1994) has identified four common errors of slippery slope thinking which all have the same feature in common: they are all unclear and rely on generalities to fuel the debate. The first element is that this line of reasoning fails to clearly identify what the bottom point of the slippery slope is or what it is that people fear most about the outcome of legalised euthanasia. Secondly, the cause of the slide down the slippery slope from the current situation to the predicted bad outcome is not identified. There are often obtuse references to impending wealth on the part of those who may benefit from the death of another, but this argument fails to clearly identify what the actual event is or has been.

The third flaw in the argument is that it does not demonstrate the badness of the outcome. As seen in the previous argument, the bad outcome is never made clear. Pabst Battin says 'if the bad outcome is simply that any individual is recognised to have the right to die while the integrity of the decision to live or die were safeguarded, it is by no means clear that this would be a bad thing'.

There is another well known argument that is used to fuel the euthanasia debate. For those opposed to the practice of euthanasia, the discussion of the Nazi practices during the Second World War inevitably enters into the discussion as an example of how the slippery slope has existed in the past. Rachels (1986) offers a very clear and sound explanation for how this argument started and how it has been maintained for almost fifty years. The atrocities committed by the Nazis during the war against Jews and other 'undesirables' as they were then known, have been widely reported. The Nuremberg trials convicted several doctors of war crimes and of the atrocities committed during Hitler's regime.

The historical link between euthanasia and Nazism has been credited to an American doctor, Leo Alexander, who identified an opportunity to use Nazi atrocities as a way to discredit euthanasia. He started by crafting a story that showed the Nazis as first using euthanasia as a way to assist the terminally ill. Once the first step was taken, so we are led to believe, the downward slide on the slippery slope was very easy: morals were abandoned and mass killing became easy. An article he wrote for the *New England Journal of Medicine* in 1949 said:

Whatever proportions [Nazi] crimes finally assumed, it became evident to all who investigated them that they started from small beginnings. The beginnings at first were merely a subtle shift in emphasis in the basic attitude of physicians. It started with the acceptance of the attitude, basic in the euthanasia movement, that there is such a thing as life not worthy to be lived. This attitude in its early stages concerned itself with the severely and chronically sick. Gradually the sphere of those to be included in this category was enlarged to encompass the socially unproductive, the ideologically unwanted, the racially unwanted and finally all non-Germans. But it is important to realise that the infinitely small wedged-in lever from which this entire trend of mind received its impetus was the attitude toward the non-rehabilitable sick. (quoted from Rachels, 1986)

Rachels offers us this rich historical account to set the stage for the other arguments that should counterbalance the Nazi argument to euthanasia. An implausible belief to be challenged is that Hitler and those involved in mass murders were initially altruistic individuals whose 'compassion' led them to kill out of a sense of mercy and that it was this compassion that allowed them to carry on to commit the atrocities that have haunted us to the present day. Even the most uninformed reader would have difficulty believing that compassion could be so boundless, particularly knowing how much cruelty was involved in the commission of these acts.

The next issue to consider is that, in the context of this discussion, euthanasia is a voluntary request by a patient to bring about his or her death. Brock (1994) identifies the need for opponents of euthanasia to consider that the values that are consistent with voluntary euthanasia are in no way consistent with the involuntary killing that defined the euthanasia of Hitler's concentration camps. In Nazi Germany, there was never an element of consent on the part of the concentration camp victims. There was no choice involved, no permission given. People were killed in the name of achieving the purity of the Aryan race. Rachels (1986) noted that Hitler accepted the notion of a life not worthy to be lived, but this was not the same notion accepted by those who are in favour of euthanasia today. Hitler's version of the life not worthy to be lived was the life that could not fulfil the dream of a pure race.

One of the final considerations in this counterplan is to examine how Hitler used the word euthanasia to add an element of respectability to his plan where no respectability would otherwise be ascribed. Rachels reminds us that when an action is performed that might otherwise be condemned, one way of hiding the true nature of that action is to invest it with a positive connotation. In other words, language is deliberately misused so as to confer positive status on an abhorrent action. For Hitler, the use of the word euthanasia implied that his actions and policies were much more benign than they actually were.

Tassano (1996), in his provocative style, challenges us further. He discards the dispute that philosophers have with this argument when they suggest that in order for slippery slope thinking to occur, there must be commitment on our parts to allow progression down the slippery slope, at least further than if we had allowed the first step to be taken. He maintains that the flaw in that argument is that the sequences that are predicted by invoking the slippery slope are not always merely imagined. He maintains that there are connections of social convention or of the law between them and he believes that when legal restraints are removed, it is difficult to believe that we are not further down the slope. He maintains, however, that the slippery slope argument is not sufficient to decide any one issue – that it cannot be used on its own to refute euthanasia, for example. He exhorts us to remember that the slippery slope argument is not relevant. This is an invitation to read the many works on the subject to develop a balanced place for this argument in your own thinking.

An ethical doctrine that is closely linked with passive euthanasia or 'treatment limiting decisions' is the doctrine of double effect. A traditional Catholic doctrine, it suggests that 'one may perform an action with a bad effect – for instance the death of a person – provided one foresees but does not *intend* (my italics) the bad effect; one must be doing the act to achieve a good effect'. As there can be two results from the single action, there is a double effect, hence the name of the doctrine. The doctrine requires that four conditions are met. The action must not be intrinsically wrong. The person performing the act must intend only a good effect, not a bad one. The bad effect must not be the means of achieving the good effect. Finally, the good effect must be proportional to, or outweigh the bad effect (Pabst Battin, 1994). The House of Lords report (1993) suggests the use of the term double effect as it relates to the administration of drugs to relieve pain and suffering with the probable consequence that it will shorten someone's life, in preference to the term passive euthanasia. The concept of intention is one that will not be explored further in this chapter, but is one worth exploring in more extensive reading.

THE ROLE OF PALLIATIVE CARE

A rich tradition of palliative care has developed around the world. One of the greatest fears shared by patients and members of their families is that they will experience a painful or otherwise distressing death. It has always been the mission of palliative care to relieve the symptoms of terminal illness, including pain, breathlessness and other distressing side effects. Dame Cecily Saunders, one of the pioneering forces in the palliative care movement said in 1972, 'All those who work with dying people are anxious that what is known already should be developed and extended and that terminal care everywhere should become so good that no one need ever ask for voluntary euthanasia.' (Glover, 1990)

While there are some elements of that argument that can be supported, it is a fundamentally flawed thesis that fails to acknowledge some basic facts about the provision of palliative care and the underlying ability of an individual to choose his or her own destiny, regardless of what supports are on offer.

As a general rule, the positive value of palliative care to a majority of patients and their carers cannot be denied. The level and quality of care generally provided helps to alleviate many of the physical and psychological symptoms experienced by patients. As death is an unfamiliar experience to most people, it is likely that the treatments and support that are available to ameliorate this condition are not known to them. If a patient is part of a health system that provides good palliative care and he or she is willing to accept it, then it is possible that some of the fears that would lead to an individual wanting to die prematurely could be allayed.

The benefits of good palliative care are vast, but it is too simplistic an argument to suggest that access to palliative care is the definitive answer for all patients who are at the end of their lives. Palliative care is not a panacea and however good the care, it may not be the answer for a select group of patients who do ask for a premature end to their lives. It is worth stressing that the numbers of patients who fall into this category are small.

The argument about the provision of palliative care being the answer becomes flawed when considering that good palliative care is still not available to the majority of terminally ill patients. It is still the case that specialist palliative care is an option for a relatively small number of patients who may fit into constricted diagnostic categories which include cancer, motor neurone disease and AIDS. The willingness or ability of the palliative care community to care for many patients outside these groups is still quite limited, owing either to a lack of specialist clinical knowledge or to the recognition that other diagnoses have a much less definable prognostic period which conflicts with the time-limited period that is often set by palliative care providers. Weigands (1988-89) suggests that patients in persistent vegetative state, for instance, would fall well outside the ambit of palliative care as the perception is that they do not feel pain or necessarily experience any of the other symptoms that palliative care deals with so well.

Another flaw linked with this argument is the supposition that palliative care is so all-encompassing that it provides all of the answers to another person's suffering. Pabst Battin (1994) makes a powerful suggestion that not all pain or other distressing symptoms can be relieved by the best efforts of the palliative care community. She goes further to suggest that when that cannot occur, there are opportunities to sedate the patient into unconsciousness, thus ending the pain and symptoms. She maintains that this culminates in causing the patient's death in respect of the patient's experience. Linking in with the criteria of the proposed Medical Futility Bill, the patient has no further conscious experience and cannot experience significant communication. She finishes by saying: 'although it is always technically possible to achieve relief from pain, at least when the appropriate resources are available, the price may be functionally and practically equivalent, at least from the patient's view, to death. And this, of course, is what the issue of euthanasia is all about'.

Farsides (1996) suggests that there may be a feeling of failure on the part of palliative care providers if a patient requests euthanasia. Those providing palliative care have carved a niche for themselves as carers rather than curers, which, in itself, flies in the face of the traditional medical model. What the carers may not have reconciled themselves to, she argues, is an acceptance of the way someone dies. At the bottom of a request for euthanasia is a perceived acknowledgement of failure on the part of the carers. How 'successful' a death is validates their ability. Far from validating a carer's needs, Farsides suggests that a request for euthanasia is an expression of personal autonomy. Regardless of the quality of care and the resources available to provide it, there are some individuals who are unable to countenance the thought of living with a deteriorating mind and/or body. They may feel that being cared for is a burden with which they are unable to live. The argument is further and more powerfully developed by Ronald Dworkin (1993) who has suggested that a failure to acknowledge that someone wishes to die, or to die in a way that others approve, but that is a horrifying contradiction of the patient's life is 'a devastating, odious form of tyranny'.

The ethical principles that have been under discussion have also found companion arguments that are commonly used to confirm the benefits or failings of euthanasia. When argued in the courts, there are arguments that arise time after time, almost as the practical disagreements that follow the theoretical. One such issue is the sanctity of life. Dworkin identifies the principle as the intrinsic value of life above all else. He says that it is the distinction between the intrinsic value of human life and its personal value for the patient that explains why so many people think euthanasia is wrong in all circumstances. It is at the heart of all religious arguments. John Locke, the philosopher, said that 'human life was not the property of the person living that life, who is just a tenant, but of God'. Dworkin goes on to say that the conviction of the sanctity of life provides a powerful emotional basis for euthanasia. Conclusions made by a working party on euthanasia and clinical practice in 1982 identified that 'men are not like other animals, they are spirit as well as flesh. Their lives are sustained by the power of God and at his will and, being spirit, a man can either consent or rebel against that will... The valuation of human life is clearly religious... a basically religious valuation of human life has preserved our homicide laws and has hitherto preserved us' (Linacre, 1984). Is this a naive argument? Does opposition to euthanasia seem outmoded simply because it is a product of Christian teaching as James Rachels suggests? Does this mean that the non-religious person could find fault with the sanctity of life argument? Dworkin maintains that atheists may feel that human life has intrinsic value. This may identify the foundations for a profound argument that sanctity of life or the intrinsic value of life, whether secular or religious, are arguments for, rather than against euthanasia.

Another argument that is put forth when considering the enormity of the subject of euthanasia is the 'best interests' argument. When thinking about other ethical principles that arise in palliative care, there are opportunities to examine the role of paternalism in decision making. Dworkin (1993) expands on this when suggesting that those who are opposed to euthanasia are opposed on paternalistic grounds – the decisions they make are in the best interests of the patient. It is these individuals who know about the interests of the patient better than the patient. The problem with the best interests argument is that it is difficult to tell in whose best interests such decisions are made. The best interests argument has had a thorough airing in the British courts as, particularly, the House of Lords struggled with the decision to discontinue food and fluids for Tony Bland in Airedale NHS Trust v Bland (1993).

A healthcare professional or family member may feel that a patient does not need to know their diagnosis or prognosis and the issue of 'truth-telling' becomes enmeshed in the best interests argument. Faulder (1985) adds this to the list of ethical considerations where it is known as the principle of veracity. Veracity is closely linked with trust and if this perceived as being abused by the patient, it is easy to see how the clinician-patient relationship could be eroded. 'Tell them what they need to know' and, particularly if it is something of a technical nature, assume they will never understand it, seems to be a prevailing theme in paternalistic arguments – perhaps not lie-telling but at the least economies with the truth and with information fall into this category. It is often not clear whether this is an altruistic approach of genuinely wanting to spare the patient the anxiety of dealing with the truth, or whether it is an issue of control. This is an area to explore and reflect upon further.

A third argument is the substituted judgement test, used often in the courts when attempting to make decisions about the withdrawal of treatment for an incompetent patient and in some cases on behalf of a competent patient. Unless the courts have a specific directive from a patient such as an advance directive or 'living will' outlining definite choices regarding treatment, they will as they did in the case of Karen Quinlan, attempt 'to don the mental mantle' of the patient. In other words, the courts will attempt to identify through previous conversations and from a patient's former attitude to life what they would have chosen for themselves in terms of withholding or withdrawing treatment. (70 NJ 10 In the Matter of Karen Quinlan, An Alleged Incompetent, Supreme Court of New Jersey 355 A 2d 647)

Some of the criticisms of this doctrine have been that it failed to differentiate between the competent and incompetent patient and that it inferred competence where it may not have existed (Oxman, 1989-90).

Advance directives have been developed to assist clinicians and the courts to more clearly identify the wishes of a patient should they become mentally incompetent for whatever reason. In March 1995, the Law Commission published a report on mental incapacity recommending urgent reform in this area of the law where it suggested that there should be statutory rules to clarify the law about the legality of advance statements or directives. It should be noted that advance directives themselves are not necessarily dynamic documents. The individual who signs such a document does so knowing what technology and treatments are available at the time. An advance directive may 'expire' technologically owing to advances in the field and it is possible that there may be an efficacious treatment available later than was thought at the time of signing the document. It is for that reason that those who sign such documents should be vigilant about reviewing and revising their wishes on a regular basis. Following the groundwork laid by the most important legal case of this kind in the United States, the Karen Quinlan case cited earlier, a second PVS case refined the law regarding advance directives in the United States. Cruzan v Director, Missouri Department of Health played a very important role in assisting each State to make provisions for advance directives. Congress adopted a law in 1990 requiring all federally supported hospitals to inform any admitted patient of each state's advance directive laws (as quoted in Dworkin 1993).

Unlike the US, physicians in England and Wales may find the directives 'helpful', but they are not bound to obey them (Spiers, 1997). Spiers identifies that they represent a beginning to allowing a patient with specific wishes to reject treatment when they are no longer capable of articulating those wishes. There are real concerns that, at least in Britain and in Canada, a doctor is not duty-bound under the law to respect a patient's wishes in an advanced directive and therefore, a reliance on professional judgement that borders on the paternalistic comes into play. Tassano (1995) suggests that the principal effect of these 'living wills' is to make it easier for doctors to withdraw treatments when they consider it appropriate, supporting the notion of paternalism.

The balance of all of these arguments is critical when examining the essential premises for discussions around euthanasia. Rights are central to the euthanasia debate. Rights can be moral or legal. A moral right must be proved to be grounded in universally applied principles and is intrinsically good. A moral right is not necessarily enforceable, although if sufficient public pressure exists, this may influence the drafting of legislation to protect that right. A legal right does not have to be supported by a moral principle – the only concern for the courts is what is right and what is wrong in the law (Faulder, 1985).

Do we have the right to ask for euthanasia? Who should be making these decisions? Should they continue to be discussed in the courts as criminal charges? Should these decisions be made only by health professionals? Should there be panels like those proposed in The Netherlands which will take the decisions out of the courts and place them in the hands of those who are 'at the coalface'?

These questions and many more are very real. To be comfortable and credible when questions about the end of life are being discussed, one should be aware of all of the elements contained in the most often quoted principles. This chapter offers only a birds-eye view of the richness of the subject and will certainly not fully inform any argument. Your role is to research and practice your arguments and beliefs. There is no right or wrong in this arena: this is your stage.

References

American Medical Association. (1996). Code of Medical Ethics: Physician-assisted suicide. *Bulletin of Medical Ethics*, June, p6.

Beauchamp T and Childress J. (1979). *Principles of Biomedical Ethics*. Oxford: Oxford University Press.

Brock D. (1994). *Life and Death: Philosophical essays in biomedical ethics*. Cambridge: Cambridge University Press.

Care in the courts, Editorial. *The Times*, Sunday 11 March 1995. Quoting Virginia Bottomley.

Dworkin R. (1993). *Life's Dominion*. London: Harper Collins.

Farsides C. (1996). Euthanasia: Failure or autonomy? *International Journal of Palliative Nursing*, 2(2), 102-5.

Faulder C. (1985). W*hose Body Is It: The troubling issue of informed consent*. London: Virago Press.

Glover J. (1977). *Causing Death and Saving Lives*. London: Penguin Books.

Gormally L. (ed.) (1994). *Euthanasia, Clinical Practice and the Law*. London: Linacre Centre.

House of Lords. (1993). *Report of the Select Committee on Medical Ethics*. Vol. 1.

Lamb D. (1985). *Death, Brain Death and Ethics*. London:

Law Commission Report. (1995). *Mental Incapacity*. No. 231. London: HMSO.

Linacre Centre. (1984). *Report of a Working Party on Euthanasia: Trends, principles and alternatives*. London: Linacre Centre.

Mason JK and Mulligan D. (1996). Euthanasia by stages. *Lancet*, 347, 810-11.

Oxman M. (1989-90). The encouragement of empathy: Just decision making for incompetent patients. *The Journal of Law and Health*, 3(2), 189-217.

Pabst Battin M. (1994). *The Least Worst Death*. Oxford: Oxford University Press.

Rachels J. (1986). *The End of Life: Euthanasia and morality*. Oxford: Oxford University Press.

Roy D and Rapin H. (1995). Regarding euthanasia. *European Journal of Palliative Medicine*, 1(1), 57-9.

Sheldon T. (1997). Dutch relax euthanasia rules. *BMJ*, 314, 325.

Spanjer M. (1996). Dutch euthanasia society solicits complaints. *Lancet*, 348, 954.

Spiers J. (1997). *Who Owns Our Bodies: Making moral choices in healthcare*. Abingdon: Radcliffe Medical Press.

Tassano F. (1995). *The Power of Life and Death: A critique of medical tyranny*. London: Gerald Duckworth Ltd.

Weigands W. (1988-89). Has the time come for Doctor Death: Should physician-assisted suicide be legalised? *Journal of Health and Law*, 7, 321-50.

Wilkes E. (1994). On withholding nutrition and hydration in the terminally ill: Has palliative medicine gone too far? A Commentary. *J Med Ethics*, 20, 144.

Zinn C. (1997). Australia repeals world's first right-to-die law. *The Guardian*, Tuesday 25 March.

Sincere thanks to the St. Gemma's Hospice library for their assistance in loaning me out-of-print materials.

CHAPTER SEVEN

Teaching ethics in the practice setting

Rachel Burman

Dr Rachel Burman MRCP, MA is a Consultant in Palliative Medicine and Director of Education at Trinity Hospice, London. A training in hospital medicine preceded her specialist training in palliative medicine and is the background to a particular interest in generic palliative care. A continued interest in ethical issues resulted in the completion of an MA in Medical Law and Ethics from the Centre of Medical Law and Ethics, London University. She is regularly involved in teaching the topic to multiprofessional groups and undergraduate medical students.

The importance of clinical ethics should not now be in doubt. It is based on the four basic *prima facie* principles of beneficence, non-maleficence, autonomy and justice. The expansion of the subject comes in the context of enormous advancements in the practice of medicine, both technological and scientific. With this has come an increasing public and professional interest in its implications. The issue of limited resources and the open discussion of the allocation of these resources is now a matter of repeated public interest. With this must also come a responsibility for healthcare workers to be educated in these principles and their application to the clinical setting.

Historically, the discussion of ethical issues in medicine took place primarily within the medical profession itself. The first and most often quoted ethical code, the Hippocratic Oath, still the basis of the ethical code by which doctors are taught to practice, is the teaching of a physician, Hippocrates. But medical ethics is not a purely medical discipline; it is the fusion or merging of many disciplines – behavioural sciences, law, theology and philosophy as well as medicine. Thus modern bioethics is the synthesis of a multidisciplinary, pluralist approach. Arguably therefore, it seems it is also best discussed and taught to multidisciplinary groups. An understanding of the principles of bioethics is vital to all those involved in the education of health workers to ensure that their own practice is defensible and justified ethically. It is also equally important in their role as teachers influencing healthcare workers in their learning and decision making, so that subsequently any decisions they should then make concerning their clients take on a justifiable ethical dimension.

Palliative care has at its core not only the discipline of rigorous control of pain and other symptoms but also the need for patient centered communication, the holistic care of the patient and their family, consideration of the needs of the patient in the context of their family, consideration of any advanced wishes of the patient, and respect for the spiritual or religious beliefs of the patient and their family. Underpinning this must be an ethical framework on which to base decision making. Since its inception, palliative care has adopted and actively fostered the multiprofessional approach to the total holistic care of patients. This model is one which palliative care has promoted to other healthcare disciplines and this philosophy has relevance to much of healthcare generally. Palliative care has always had interests which cut across traditional departmental and divisional lines; it has adopted novel approaches to interdepartmental and interdisciplinary programmes throughout its evolution. Palliative care is therefore well placed to again lead the field in the multidisciplinary teaching of bioethics.

The practice of palliative care takes place within the whole spectrum of clinical or practice settings. There is the more traditional model of hospice based work, this inpatient setting also offering an outreach facility through a home care team which works with the patient and their family in the setting of their own home. In this practice setting there is close liaison with colleagues in district nursing and general practice. More recently there has been the development of hospital based support teams. Teams of nurses, doctors and hospital social workers in conjunction with colleagues in the physiotherapy and occupational health departments, provide a palliative care input to patients whilst they are in hospital. The patients seen in hospital may be at an earlier stage in their illness than that traditionally seen in the hospice setting and the role of the team in facilitating information about the prognosis is essential. Patients in this practice setting may find that their first point of contact with palliative care is around the discussion of the transition of their care from a curative to a palliative approach. There are particular ethical issues surrounding this. The palliative care team may be called upon to become involved in the discussion surrounding the issues of withdrawing treatment from a patient in the acute hospital setting.

The day to day practice of palliative care continually involves the confrontation and discussion of ethical issues which require a pragmatic resolution in the work of all healthcare professionals. Daily decisions about the ongoing treatment of terminally ill patients and the degree of active intervention which should be undertaken are discussed and decided. The respect for a patient's autonomy is particularly challenging in the context of a request for euthanasia from either a patient or a carer. The need to sensitively handle a carer's or patient's request for disclosure or non-disclosure of information, particularly concerning length of prognosis, is a constant dilemma. The different philosophical approaches to the issues which surround death and dying encountered when practising in a multifaith society are all routine issues for a palliative care team. This team has always included not only nurses and doctors but also social workers, counsellors and chaplains.

It is therefore universally accepted that the teaching of ethics is desirable. The next concern is, how is this to be most effectively achieved? All the professional bodies responsible for the content of courses for healthcare workers agree that an ethics component is indicated but are not explicit about what it should contain. The training of doctors is overseen by the General Medical Council; it has decreed that ethics teaching should be part of the core curriculum for medical students but leaves the content and organization of the teaching to the individual medical schools (GMC, 1993). Furthermore there is a lack of staff with any training in the subject available to teach it. Grant et al (1989) and later Seedhouse (1991) observe that courses are taught by people with no philosophical background, and insufficient time is allowed for proper analysis of ethical problems. The emphasis should be on allowing sensitive listening to and discussion of experiences and ethical dilemmas, with philosophers and clinicians facilitating. On average the length of time allocated to the subject is 0.1% of all undergraduate teaching. Self (1988) confirms that often the teaching of ethics is didactic, focussing on curriculum content and teaching methods to the exclusion of the contribution that the medical students themselves can make. A number of studies have looked at the level of ethical awareness of various groups prior to their respective trainings. Self (1988) showed a resistance from some medical students to ethical teaching, fearing that in a multicultural society all belief structures should be afforded equal respect and that formal instruction in ethics would represent a form of indoctrination.

Grundstein-Amando (1992) found differences between the various healthcare professional groups. Nursing students were more generally concerned to motivate their ethical reasoning with the fundamental of caring whilst medical students were more motivated by the concepts of patients' rights. Other researchers have looked at other rationales for the apparent differences in various groups. Gilligan (1982) postulates that there is a difference based on gender, with females more often seeing morality in the context of particular relationships, whilst men sublimate this to a view of impartiality and justice. Kolhberg (1971) disagrees with this construct, arguing that personal morality has little to do with gender and more to do with the individual. Nolan and Smith (1995) showed that medical students do not come to their training devoid of material which could form the basis of a program of ethics teaching. On the contrary, they have already derived much from relevant reading and work experience prior to attending medical school. Another finding of this study was that the majority of students considered the teaching of ethics to be important, and that they would like this teaching to be practically based.

There is a growing call for ethical teaching in the undergraduate curriculum, but there is not the corresponding attention to the subject in the clinical training years. Recent studies here and in the

USA have shown that practising physicians felt their education in treating disease was excellent whilst areas such as healthcare resource allocation and ethical issues were poorly covered. These studies have highlighted barriers to change such as departmentalization of the medical school, lack of leadership and lack of faculty development. Despite recognition of the need for change there has been little substantial curricular innovation and then only in the preclinical years. Fleischman and Arras (1987) observe that the *ad hoc* discussion of cases without reference to philosophical principles tends to yield aimless, ungrounded speech; abstract theoretical discussion of philosophical doctrines often proves irrelevant to the concrete and urgent concerns of the physician.

The challenge in teaching medical students is to integrate philosophical theory with concrete clinical case material. The special perspective of the family practitioner is evaluated in the paper by Stevens et al (1993). This is an example of case-based teaching, in the primary care setting. A sessional course meets weekly for 10 sessions to discuss ethical topics such as truth-telling, informed consent and autonomy. Then the family practitioner presents a real case from their practice and explains it up until the ethical decision is made. At this point the group of students is encouraged to discuss what decision they would come to. The goals of these sessions are to develop the students' ability to define the issues and think about possible resolutions in a way that also helps them analyse their own moral reasoning. These classes include not only medical students but also students of nursing, pharmacy and physiotherapy. The students reported that representations of different professional disciplines enriched the group, that the use of everyday clinical cases was much more instructive than the use of more highly published dilemmas, and that exposure to the family practitioner allowed them to understand context-sensitive care.

One model which has tried to cross the disciplines in its approach to the teaching of ethics in the clinical years is in practice at UCLA medical school (Slavin et al, 1995). In the third year of study (the first clinical year), the students follow a longitudinal program of simulated practice sessions where they meet one or two new patients and follow up three or four patients. These simulations use taped phone calls and video consultations with patients. The content of these encounters is built around 25 patient scenarios most commonly seen by a hospital doctor and includes issues of ethics and resource allocation. Thus the students follow the course of these patients and in ordering their tests and discussing their management gain experience of evidence-based medicine. In the small discussion groups through the year they become confident in the reasoning needed to explore the ethical issues confronted in clinical practice. This model of training has the benefit of integrating the ethical teaching into the clinical situation in a realistic and therefore accessible way for the students, who report it as being much easier to see the relevance of this subject to their work as doctors. This contrasts with the complaints of other students that ethical teaching in their experience is didactic and too philosophical.

Joseph and Conrad (1983) have published work looking specifically at the issue of ethical training in social work. They rightly argue that for the effective working of the multiprofessional team, a social worker must feel confident to participate in the team's discussion of ethical dilemmas. They also point out that, to date, there has been little formal training available. The absence of this ability will in time lead to abdication of moral power and diminished professional responsibility. Further work by Joseph and Conrad identifies some predictors of social work influence in this area. They emphasise the ethical dilemmas not only pertaining to the client but also the interprofessional issues of skill mix, information sharing and role clarity. They also have the courage to challenge the quality of the people currently responsible for what teaching there is. They highlight that there is not necessarily adequate preparation of the professionals given this responsibility.

Several people (Leavitt, 1996; Scott, 1996) have written that the nursing body is the one best able to move into the arena of bioethics. They argue that nurses are equipped with a large amount of clinical experience and are the professionals most likely to deal with the day to day manifestations of ethical dilemmas and the patients and families they affect. There has long been a tradition of nurses putting themselves forward as the patient and family advocate. This tradition sits well with the basic principle of respect for patient autonomy. Nurses also, more often than other healthcare workers, return to structured further study following a period of clinical work. The scene is therefore set for the synthesis of practical experience and more formal philosophical thought and teaching which is agreed to be the necessary basis for bioethics. This discipline is about the personal side of healthcare as it deals with settling or preempting possible conflicts between professional medical expertise and the autonomy of the patient and their family. Some would argue that nurses are the best placed for this role, once trained in ethical principles and reasoning.

A recent development in the application of medical ethics is the formation of ethical committees (Dunn and Hansen-Flaschen, 1994), and most recently the concept of an ethical consultation with an ethicist. This practice is still confined to the USA and Canada where many of the larger hospitals have resident ethicists on their staff. Ethical committees in this context are not the same as those in this country which are solely for the consideration of research protocols submitted in the hospital setting. In the USA, ethics committees are commonplace in healthcare institutions. They have a multiprofessional membership, with equal numbers of physicians and nurses along with members who are lawyers, clergy, social workers, administrators, members of the public and patients. The process of membership selection is not always clearly set out but is based on some past experience and ability to contribute to the committee. These committees normally have a three-fold purpose: the recommendation of policy, a role in education of the healthcare professionals in the hospital, and a role in specific case consultations. Many of the policies developed over the last ten years regarding such issues as Do-Not-Resuscitate orders and the usefulness of advanced directives have been derived by the consensus of such committees. However, the existence of such committees and the formulation of their policies does not translate directly into the understanding of the clinicians themselves. There is often a gap between prevailing guidelines and the knowledge and views of many doctors and nurses. Following the creation of such policies, committees must create strategies to influence the attitudes of the clinicians.

The role of education is pivotal to the successful implementation of these policies. An increase in healthcare practitioners' awareness of and ability to assess ethical problems will eventually ease the burden of the educational component to the work of the committee. Those committees that monitor the impact of the teaching on new professionals will also be able to help new schools and programs. They will also be able to influence the content of other modules being developed in other settings.

Specific case consultations are generally carried out by a team of some members of the committee. Each team within the committee takes it in turns to be on call for a two week period. There may be an addition to the team, based on a needs assessment and the area of expertise required. For example in an issue concerning maternal-child matters a member from the obstetrics team would be co-opted. On occasions, new members of the committee attend to gain experience as observers. A request for a consultation may be made by a nurse, doctor or social worker for example, or by the family or patient themselves. Most of the consultations take place within 48 hours of the referral being made. Normally a team leader is appointed and they will conduct the consultation.

The first objective is to delineate the problems of the particular case which are often the results of a lack of communication between the healthcare team and the patient. The emphasis is not on the ethical knowledge of the team but more on what the team can enable or mediate for the patient and their family.

There are a number of questions which need to be addressed by the team. These include: is the patient competent, what is the belief system of the patient, are there any particular requests or mandates the patient wants to make, what, if any, are the conflicts between the healthcare professional and the patient?

Following this process the issues are summarised and the patient and the family make decisions which are then looked at by the team from an ethical perspective. Group consensus is usually achieved. This approach not only clarifies the values and explores the ethical dilemmas but also allows a decision to be made.

In the USA this model of ethical teaching and practice is being extended to the community setting. This committee process which started as a self educating one is now expanding its educational efforts to healthcare workers and the public more and more. It is also expanding its educational efforts increasingly to the area of healthcare resource allocation (Perlin, 1992).

In conclusion, it can be seen that all healthcare professionals, of whatever discipline, recognise a need for the inclusion of ethical reasoning into their respective trainings. It is also clear that it is pertinent particularly to the specialty of palliative care. A review of the literature has shown that what they bring even at the point of beginning their respective trainings has a bearing on the way that they most effectively learn these principles and the reasoning skills to apply them.

Some authors have rightly raised the issue of who best teaches this subject, to whom and with whom. The literature supports the principle of interdisciplinary teaching and learning, suggesting that the cross fertilization of this approach is beneficial to all. This is a concept that fits well with the teaching that takes place on other topics in the specialty of palliative medicine and can happily be adopted and built upon by all healthcare workers in the discipline.

It has been shown that the quality of the teaching given to students in itself is necessary to validate the subject of medical ethics and to emphasise its obvious importance. Whilst it seems to be universally accepted that the theoretical teaching of medical ethics has a place early on in the curricula of all healthcare workers, the teaching is often didactic in nature. The need for it to be contextualised in the clinical setting with the use of case histories is not always recognised and the teaching is therefore less effective. Not surprisingly the teaching and unfortunately the subject itself are then valued less highly. This is especially true of the experience of medical students at present. The evolution of ethical committees and the formalizing of the ethical consultation underlines that the best practice is that of multiprofessional working.

Palliative care in this country is already well established in its practice of multiprofessional team working and should the more easily adopt this effective approach when dealing with ethical dilemmas faced and teaching these principles to other healthcare workers either in training or already practising.

References

Dunn AP, Hansen-Flaschen J. (1994). Framework for analysing an ethical problem and conducting an ethical consultation. *Seminars for Nurse Managers*, 2, 27-30.

Fleischman AR, Arras J. (1987). Teaching medical ethics in perinatology. *Clin Perinatol*, 14, 395-402.

Gilligan C. (1982). *In a Different Voice*. Cambridge, Massachusetts: Harvard University Press.

GMC. (1993). *Tomorrow's Doctors: Recommendations for Undergraduate Medical Education*. London: General Medical Council.

Grant VJ et al. (1989). Advanced medical ethics for fifth year students. *J Med Ethics*, 15, 200-2.

Grundstein-Amando R. (1992). Differences in ethical decision making processes among nurses and doctors. *J Adv Nurs*, 17, 129-37.

Joseph MV, Conrad AP. (1983). Teaching social work ethics for contemporary practice: an effective evaluation. *Journal for Social Work Education*, 19, 59-68.

Kolhberg L. (1971). From is to ought. In: Mitchel T. (ed.) *Cognitive Development and Epistemology*. New York: Academic Press.

Leavitt FJ. (1996). Educating nurses for their role in bioethics. *Nursing Ethics*, 3, 40-51.

Nolan PW, Smith J. (1995). Ethical awareness in first year medical, dental and nursing students. *Int J Stud*, 32(5), 506-17.

Perlin T. (1992). *Clinical Medical Ethics Cases in Practice*. Boston: Little, Brown and Co.

Scott PA. (1996). Ethics education and nursing practice. *Nursing Ethics*, 4, 53-6.

Seedhouse D. (1991). healthcare ethics teaching for medical students. *Med Educ*, 25, 230-7.

Self DJ. (1988). The pedogogy of two different approaches to humanistic medical education; cognitive vs affective. *Theoret Med*, 9, 227-36.

Slavin SJ, Wilkes MS, Usatine MD. (1995). Doctoring III: innovations in education in the clinical years. *Academic Medicine*, 70, 1091-5.

Stevens NG, McCormick TR. (1993). Bringing the special perspective of the family physician to the teaching of clinical ethics. *J Am Board Fam Pract*, 7, 38-43.